ALIVE WITH LIFE

Other books by Gary Epler:

You're the Boss: Manage Your Disease
BOOP: You're the Boss
Asthma: You're the Boss
Food: You're the Boss
Fuel for Life: Level-10 Energy

ALIVE WITH LIFE

A MEDICAL DOCTOR'S GUIDE TO LIVE YOUR BEST LIFE

GARY R. EPLER, M.D.

Waterside Press

Printed in the United States of America

First Printing, 2018

ISBN-13: 978-1-939116-58-1 print edition
ISBN-13: 978-1-939116-59-8 ebook edition

Waterside Productions
2055 Oxford Ave
Cardiff, CA 92007
www.waterside.com

*This book is dedicated to people everywhere
who live a healthy and happy life on their own terms.*

And to

*My beautiful wife, Joan, whose life is filled with love and happiness,
and my two sons Greg and Brett*

ACKNOWLEDGMENTS

My thanks go to the many people whose insights have helped develop the material for this book. My special thanks goes to Professor Marty Seligman at UPenn for his ground-breaking development of well-being concepts. My thanks goes to Professor Mihaly Csikszentmihalyi at the University of Chicago for his insight into the nine elements of flow, and to Professor Kevin Flanigan of West Chester University in Pennsylvania for his enjoyment and knowledge of English words. Thanks to Dr. Lissa Rankin for her insight about self-healing in her book *Mind Over Medicine*. My thanks to Elizabeth Dunn and Michael Norton for their research about giving away money, and Kristin Neff, professor at the University of Texas at Austin, for her profound insights into self-compassion. Thanks to Robert Emmons and Michael McCullough for their insight and study of the beneficial effects of gratitude, and to Professor Peter M. Vishton at William and Mary for his "Outsmart Yourself" lecture series. Thanks to Mike Michalowicz for his insights of eliminating financial stress in his book, *Profit First*, and to Oren Klaff for his perception into the "crock brain" for successful sales in his book, *Pitch Anything*. Additional individuals to thank include Professor Robert Garland for his insight into daily life during ancient times, decision making by Professor Ryan Hamilton, and 5000 years of Chinese history by Professor Kenneth J. Hammond. Thanks to Scott Molgard, elite master personal trainer, for his enthusiastic support and contribution. Thanks to Kay McManus and Nichole Bernier for their editing expertise.

CONTENTS

Alive with Life
A Medical Doctor's Guide to Live Your Best Life

1. Who Knew Life Could Be So Easy: Live Life with Pizzazz 1
2. Create Happiness for the Zest of Life 5
3. Be Alive, Engage in Life 10
4. Build Meaning into Your Life for an Improved World 13
5. Accomplishments Propel You to Well-Being. 22
6. Sustainable Positive Social Interaction 25
7. You Gotta Love Life: The First of Ten Health Practices. 31
8. Nutrition Is a Lifestyle, Not a Diet 35
9. Sleep: You Need Eight Hours 66
10. Exercise: You Might Meet Your Spouse. 75
11. Learn Something New for a Creative Life 89
12. Alpha-Brainwave Meditation Time 99
13. Compassion for Peace of Mind 112
14. Gratitude. 115
15. You Can Learn Self-Healing 117
16. Be Your True Self 136
17. Optimism 143
18. You're the Boss: Manage Your Disease 145
19. Live to 140 169
20. Level-10 Energy Is Fuel for Life 177
21. People-Centered Leadership 186
22. Hard Work and American Entrepreneurship 191
23. Business One-Liners 211
24. How to Use This Book 216

CHAPTER 1
WHO KNEW LIFE
COULD BE SO EASY:
LIVE LIFE WITH PIZZAZZ

Imagine what life is like when you feel good all the time. Think for a moment about a *best day*. I'm talking about a day when you felt spectacular just being yourself on top of the world – healthy, happy, and at ease with others.

You don't need to imagine it any longer. This is all possible by making it happen yourself. Those wonderful days you love to have – everything goes well, nothing bothers you, you can accomplish anything. You're alive with energy. You're alert. Your eyes are open. Your mind is working. You don't see problems. You see solutions. Your mind is generating positive thoughts. You talk to people. People talk to you. You listen to people. People listen to you. You make money. You're energized by your work. You help people. People help you. You're forgiving. You're grateful. Your senses are engaged. You hear the birds. You see the flowers. You feel the softness. You smell the sweet perfume. You taste food. You're creative. You enjoy life.

How can you live a healthy and sparkling life filled with such wonderful days? By learning and implementing five components of well-being and ten health practices. The outcome will be being alive with energy and able to endure life's insults and injuries with grace.

The concept of well-being is something to strive for throughout our lives. What does "well-being" mean? It's defined as the state of being happy and healthy – the same as joie de vivre, vigor, and vitality.

Dr. Martin Seligman, at the University of Pennsylvania, developed the five-component theory of well-being, one of the most significant developments in psychology since the beginning of the discipline.

Happiness is the first component. Feeling good, optimistic, and happy is an integral part of a successful, fulfilling life. Set up your day with a positive outlook to attain as much happiness as possible.

Being engaged in life is the second component. This means experiencing the current moment. It means experiencing conversations in an ongoing continuous manner. It means knowing what you are doing, what you want, and where you're going at all times.

Finding meaning in your life is another component. Do something that's bigger than yourself. Help a person or support a business or the community without receiving anything in return.

The fourth component is fundamental to our well-being. It's **accomplishment.** Set your life up so that you achieve continuous accomplishments. These can be small daily accomplishments or long-term big accomplishments. Savor the time and feeling when you've accomplished a task.

Positive social interaction is the final component. Talk to people in a positive way so that your comments cause a positive feeling in the person you are talking to. This can be a self-renewing trait as you will receive positive feelings in return that will last the day.

Score your profile number for each of these five well-being performance measures on a scale of one to ten. Your number will vary over time. You need to strive to reach eight to ten and enjoy being there. If you're a six, try improving the score. If you're five or below, you need work. You need to spend time exploring the reasons and develop a plan to move up the scale. Improve your low scores by understanding and applying one or more of the ten health practices.

———

Let's look at health practices.

Positive health practices have been known for thousands of years. We've known about most of them since childhood. The remedy and breakthrough for a wonderful life is implementation of these practices in a sustainable manner. Having a coach to remind you to incorporate these practices into your daily life is a good way to do this, but too unrealistic for most people. Learn to be your own coach.

Although you've been told about several of these health practices since grade school and are reminded of them by the media on a daily basis, it's the *combination* of these ten practices that is powerful.

Love life is the first of the ten. Life is to be enjoyed. Look forward to the day and anticipate a great day. You're going to have positive things happen throughout the day and night. Cherish and enjoy them.

The next three are daily lifestyle practices: **eat healthy, nutritious food; get eight hours of sleep**; and **exercise continuously for one hour.**

Learn something new may seem like an unusual health practice, but this fifth one can provide a huge boost of energy and sense of accomplishment. Learn something unrelated to your work – the further away from your familiar interests, the better.

The sixth practice is **create alpha-brainwave meditation time.** This is daydreaming. The benefits include feeling good, decreasing stress, balancing brain activities, and increasing the longevity of the telomeres at the end of the chromosomes for longer cell life. Make meditation a part of your day, and it doesn't have to be traditional sitting and repeating a mantra meditation. It can be eyes-open. Alpha-brainwave time can become a part of your day without even realizing it.

The next two are **have compassion** and **be grateful.** Self-esteem will let you down, but compassion for yourself will always help. Have compassion for others. It'll make you feel good. It's so important to be grateful for what we have. This grounds us and prevents us from thinking too much about ourselves and from feeling entitled.

The penultimate practice can save your life. It's **self-healing.** Using the power of our mind can result in the healing of injuries and illness from simple bumps to complex dysfunctional disease. You can *learn* self-healing.

The final practice may take time, but it's **be your true self.** Once you totally become your true self, you will have an immense feeling of freedom. This includes freedom from criticism, from insult, from disappointment, and from failure. You will no longer use blame, excuses, criticism, or complaints.

How to use this book? Learn about these fifteen elements from the in-depth discussion in each chapter. When you're having a bad day or unable to bounce back from an insult or injury, refer to these pages for a quick reference and put in place one or more of them that will solve the issue. Reread the chapter if the reminder is not sufficient. Using one or more of these fifteen elements will help you address the problem at hand and return you to a state of having a good day.

CHAPTER 2
CREATE HAPPINESS FOR THE ZEST OF LIFE

People want to be happy. It's one of the most important sought-after ingredients of life. Everyone knows what happiness is – the feeling of joy. It puts a smile on your face. It feels good. It's bliss. It can last for a fleeting moment or for many days. It's fundamental for well-being. Create opportunities for happiness through engaging in the day, through experiences, through accomplishments, and through positive social interaction.

Genetics accounts for 50 percent of your happiness level. Look at babies. You can determine their lifetime level of happiness by simple observation. Some are smiling and active. Others are irritable and nervous.

About 10 percent of happiness comes from life events such as getting married, getting a raise, or buying a house. These wonderful occasions provide a new level of happiness; however, their effects are usually fleeting, lasting hours, months, or three to five years for marriage, and most people return to their baseline level of happiness over time.

The good news is that you're in charge of the remaining 40 percent happiness level. It's your behavior and you can manage it. People who sustain a high level of happiness focus on what's internally important to them. This means spending time doing what they enjoy – their life's calling, their passion, spending time with family and friends, and being involved in the community. People who maintain high-level happiness live in and savor the moment.

There are several science-based actions that can provide happiness.

Music can give us a feeling of happiness. Listening to the right type of music can make us happy. It produces the feel-good neurotransmitters such as endorphins.

The brain, the body, and all the cells vibrate at differing frequencies. Some types of music will cause a paired vibration resulting in energy. This is called *entrainment,* which means matching vibration. If five pendulum clocks are all set at different starting points, within four hours, the pendulum of each clock will swing at the same time in synchronous timing. Music can also function to entrain the cyclic pattern of your brain in the same manner.

Music provides an entry point into different regions of the brain. The pitch, harmony, rhythm, and emotion components of music each reach a specific part of the brain. For example, for individuals who have an injury in a specific region, music can create a pathway for improved function. Music therapy such as choral singing and rhythmic body movements can improve muscle coordination and behavioral function in Parkinson's disease.

Music can change the brain and create plasticity, which means new brain-cell neuropathway growth. After several weeks of learning to play the piano, the region of the brain involved in this activity becomes larger and more connected. Learning this new skill has rewired the brain.

Listening to music can also remind you of past memories and enjoyable times in your life. Hearing a song that was popular during a time that you were happy, going out with your future spouse, special holiday vacation spots, or a rock concert can instantly transport you back to this happy time.

Music can provide happiness during exercise, such as running, cycling, or group activities like spinning, aerobics, Zumba, or body-pump classes. For example, a song like Bob Seger's "The Fire Inside" can provide a downbeat for the right or left foot while running on the treadmill at a certain speed. The musical beat directly provides a pathway to a specific region of the brain for improved motor efficiency and energy.

The same effect occurs among people in spin class and other aerobic classes where music is played. The first song is generally slow tempo for warm-up. The middle songs are high tempo and provide a cadence for the right and left foot; the speed can be doubled for extra work. The last song is for cool-down with a slow rhythm. Music also allows individuals in the class to create a high level of energy shared by the whole class – this is what I call "Group Level-10 Energy."

All types of music can generate a good feeling. Beethoven's Egmont Overture is an up-tempo rhythmic beat, which is usually best for providing energy. Mozart's music can provide the feeling of a soaring eagle.

Yet, people vary in their response to music. Some music will have the opposite of the expected effect. For example, a beautifully played Verdi's Requiem can completely drain energy in some people yet lift the spirits of others.

Smile for the feeling of happiness. It relates to neurolinguistics – the connection between words and action. You think of happy words, you feel happy. This works in reverse too. When you smile, the brain can be fooled because there is the connection between being happy and smiling so when you're smiling, you feel happy. Frowning will make you feel sad. Smiling will make you feel happy.

Laughter, a distinct human behavior, will also bring happiness. This is especially true if the laugh is about a positive story. Laughing at other people's expense produces negative energy.

A smile creates warm feelings, feel-good neurotransmitters, and energy. People smile when they're happy, and they feel happy when they smile. Let the body change your thinking. This is through the subconscious mind. A pencil study showed this concept. One group of people held a pencil with their teeth making a smile, and another group help the pencil with their lips making a frown. Compared to a controlled group of people who did nothing, those with the pencil smile scored happier on post tests, and those with the pencil frown scored sadder. Is this why smoking cigarettes makes people sad?

Happiness improves the immune system. Having a high happiness level results in higher productivity, a better memory, and even an improved immune system. A study measured the number of antibodies from a flu shot among a group of people and measured their happiness level. Those with the highest number of antibodies and highest functioning immune system had the highest happiness level.

In the flow. You've experienced a wonderful day where everything goes well or you're working on a project when you forget about time or surroundings. You're doing something so focused you keep going and going without distractions. I call this a "Level-10 Energy" day where you're on top of the world, nothing bothers you, and you can accomplish anything.

A large part of experiencing these wonderful days is being in the *flow,* a state of mind described by University of Chicago psychologist Mihaly Csikszentmihalyi. The fundamental idea of "flow" is that you experience true satisfaction when totally absorbed in an activity where your skill level is equally balanced with the challenge.

You will experience flow if your skills are sufficient to meet the challenge. If the challenge is greater than your skill level, you may experience frustration, fear, procrastination, and no forward motion. If your skill level is greater than the challenge, you may get bored and experience no personal or cultural growth.

When your skills and the challenge you're facing are equally balanced, you always know the next step. You have immediate feedback as you move along. You are focused on the activity with no distractions. You don't think about failure. You have no thoughts about yourself, and you don't care what other people are thinking about you.

Time becomes distorted. Either it expands – becoming ten seconds doing a triple jump at a track meet that actually takes only a second, or it contracts – becoming mere minutes working on a new discovery that actually took hours. In the end, the activity becomes enjoyable to the extent that you want to do it again because it's pleasurable and brings you happiness.

There are many examples of the feeling of flow from everyday events to life-changing activities. This can happen in a conversation with someone. If your communication skills are in balance with the other person, the conversation flows and you want to see the person again. If your skills are higher, the conversation is boring and you will leave. If your skills are lower, you will feel uncomfortable and threatened and will want to figure a way to get out of the conversation as soon as possible.

Running is another example. You are running a five-mile run in the flow and enjoying the run with no distractions, no concept of time, and no thought of failure. The skills and the challenge are in balance. Then you start running up a hill. You are no longer in balance; the challenge is greater than the skills. You get short of breath, you are in pain, you want to get it over with; it's not pleasant. You have two options for returning to balance: increase the skill or decrease the challenge. In this example, the challenge is decreased as you return to running on level ground.

This is what happens when you're in the flow. If your skills are in balance with the problem, you will work on the issue night and day. You will always know the next step, you will make automatic adjustments from the instant feedback, you will not be distracted by anything, you will not think of failure, you have no thoughts about yourself, time will be forgotten, and the enjoyment from the activity will put a smile on your face. You can't wait to share the excitement with your spouse, your friends, and the world.

If your skills are too high for the discovery or the project, you will quickly lose interest and become bored. If your skills are not enough to deal with the discovery, you will be frustrated, distracted, and nervous.

Here's what you can do. Set up your life on a day-to-day basis to balance your skills with challenges as often as possible so you can experience the pleasurable feeling of flow. There will, of course, be some situations when your skill level is not equally matched to a challenge. When this happens, you don't have to master the skill, but you do need to recognize the issue, because then you will be able to proceed with completing the challenge. It won't be easy – you'll have to work at it, and the experience won't be pleasurable, but do the work without frustration or delays, and don't feel sorry for yourself. You do not need to be in the flow twenty-four hours a day.

Take on challenges. Develop new skills. Discover new insights. Be in the flow with these challenges for the feeling of pleasure and happiness.

CHAPTER 3
BE ALIVE, ENGAGE
IN LIFE

Engagement is the second component of well-being. This means being engaged in the day, not distracted by complaining, blaming, making excuses, and being critical. It means focusing on one thing at the moment. Living in the moment. This means listening to a person, not thinking about the next thing to say or looking at your cell phone.

When you are engaged in life, you interact with people *without outside distractions.* For example, someone whose job is to check in people to a workout club can do this in one of two ways. One way is talking aimlessly on a cell phone or watching a video clip while holding the barcode register with the other hand, not looking up or acknowledging the person checking in. The other way – the engaged way – is to say good morning and over days and weeks develop an ongoing conversation. Both individuals benefit from the mutual interaction.

Every job has two parts. When you're engaged in life, you don't stop at the first part of the job – you also do the second part of the job.

I had some work done on my house last year, replacing some wood that had become worn. The workmen did a terrific job of replacing the wood, couldn't have done better; but they failed miserably at the second part of the job – cleaning up and protecting the house. They left a mess. There were scraps of wood and paint on the grass, flowers were trampled, and worse, there were deep gouges in the wood on the side of the house from the ladders.

Doing the second part of the job means you are engaged in and proud of your work and that you are committed to doing it right, not taking shortcuts. You don't make excuses and you want to give people what they need and deserve. *Being engaged is the difference between being good and being the best.*

Every job has two parts, and to be the best, you have to do both parts. A good doctor diagnoses and treats disease correctly; the best doctor does this plus has a caring nature. A spin class instructor may have a good routine and great music, but not be able to create positive social interaction during the class. A good plumber fixes your sink. The best plumber fixes your sink and doesn't trample mud on your floor and doesn't leave grease on the cabinets. Need help clearing two feet of snow from your driveway? The good snow remover removes the snow from the driveway; the best removes the snow from the driveway, doesn't plow the snow into your neighbor's yard, clears the sidewalk, and cleans the edges.

Two more examples. A good lawyer tells you about the risks; the best lawyer tells you how to manage the risks. A good human resources person tells you what the problems are; the best HR person helps you find solutions to the problems.

Look at your own work. There are always two parts. You do a good job with the first. Know the second part, complete the second part, and you will be the best.

Engage in life. Finish the last five percent of the job.

My friend Bob owns a construction company and told me the first five percent and the last five percent of building a house are the hardest. Review your experience – is he right? Yes, he is. *Finishing the last five percent of any job separates the best from the average.*

My wife, Joan, and I watched two houses being built during our Sunday morning run along our neighborhood route. They were beautiful, majestic homes. They were both built quickly during several months. However, for months after building the first house, the street sidewalk remained in disrepair from the construction, and the small strip of grass between the sidewalk and the street was mud. Several months after "finishing" the second house, the protect-the-environment straw bales were still spread throughout the street and the neighbor's lawn. On a different part of our run, the owners of another new house that was built in less than a year took two years to clean up scraps of wood and finish a tiny strip of landscaping in the front. These minor details may not bother some people, but the jobs weren't finished. And this issue occurs every day in our businesses and social lives. What about the husband who takes out the trash bag, but doesn't put in a new trash bag in the barrel, leaving this annoying job for his wife? Examples are everywhere.

My friend Scott who had been a furniture mover told me about his experiences with the last five percent. If the first moving crew only moved the big, obvious items, it took the second crew two and sometimes three times longer to find, load, and pack the last five percent of small random items. On the other hand, he said that if the first crew moved what needed to be moved including extra nuisance items, the total job took half as long and cost half as much. Scott also said that when homeowners left loose pieces scattered throughout the house in the attic and basement, it took more hours to finish this last five percent than to completely empty the entire house, resulting in higher cost to the homeowner. Completing the last five percent saves money too.

Look at your work. Do you complete the job? Do you leave tools scattered throughout the house after minor repair work? Do you clean up after making a mess fixing something? At your job, do you stop at the last five percent of the project and go home? Do you let your associates or friends finish the last five percent of the work?

Finish the job every time. You will have the satisfying feeling of doing a great job, even if no one notices, and you won't have the lingering, unsettling feeling of a job not quite finished. Second, you will be more successful in your overall work and social interactions. Do the last five percent of the job to be the best.

Be engaged in life. Live and enjoy the moment. At all times, know what you want, what you're doing, and where you're going.

CHAPTER 4
BUILD MEANING INTO
YOUR LIFE FOR AN
IMPROVED WORLD

Meaning is the third component of well-being. Do something bigger than yourself. Contribute to your family, friends, the community, or a nonprofit organization. Do something without getting something in return.

There are people who lack meaning in their lives. For example, you're having a casual conversation with someone, and the person mentions a minor complaint about their job. Before you can say anything, the person's voice fills with anger. The conversation continues with complaints about too much work, a degrading job title, and of course not enough money for all the after-hours work. Your attempt at a positive conversation is ignored.

Their complaints lead to how they ended up in this job, which then leads to a long whine about making bad choices in the past and the list of should've done this or that, could've done this or that, and if only this or that had happened. You will also hear a list of excuses based on why these bad decisions were made. The one-sided discussion deteriorates further when the ramblings turn to blaming and criticizing others.

Do you know anyone like this? A family member? A friend? A boss or coworker? People who take no self-responsibility. They blame, criticize, complain, and make excuses. They only think of themselves. They don't have meaning in their life.

There are many ways to gain meaning in your life.

Help someone. When you see people who need a little help with something minor, give them a hand. You'll feel good, and you'll give that person a boost of energy. The more you help people, the more people will help you.

My friend's son had a behavioral condition that was a variant of Asperger's syndrome. His son struggled for years and years. Afraid to be in public. Too much stimulation would send him into uncontrollable panic. Too much noise. Too many people. Too many questions.

My friend developed meaning in his life, and meaning does not necessarily mean positive happy feelings. It means doing something beyond yourself. It means committing to something without reward, without payback, and without end. My friend dedicated his life to helping his child.

The struggles with my friend's son began at birth and continued for 16 years. His son was in special classes for many years, but nothing change. Then, my friend heard about a special school located in a nearby town. The cost was prohibitive. He needed help. He was denied time and again for months and years. Yet, he persisted and with the assistance of an attorney, his son was finally accepted at age 16. It was a miracle. Within a few months, his son became a normally functioning teenager at the school, at home with his family, and in public. He also became a contributing member of society. The father is the hero of this story. The father developed meaning in his life.

Give a meaningful apology. We all make mistakes and sometimes offend or hurt others without realizing it. When this happens, give a meaningful apology. There are three components for this type of apology.

Say "I'm sorry." "It's my fault." "What can I do to make it right?"

It's about the other person, and this type of apology may result in forgiveness and a return to positive social interaction.

Volunteer. Volunteering is good for your health. Stress levels are decreased and well-being increased when people stop thinking about themselves and focus on others.

Volunteer for community activities, building parks, rehabilitation projects, or coaching. Take your next one- to two-week vacation time and volunteer internationally. Look up the top ten volunteer organizations. The list of projects is endless. There is a match for your interests – wildlife research, ancient structure restoration, marine research, healthcare, or earthquake. The enjoyment is lifelong.

Volunteering provides control over your actions. You can learn new skills and a new perspective, a new way to see the world.

You will make new connections with people and cultures. You will have ongoing positive social interactions that become self-sustaining for improved well-being. You will be part of a team and learn that people need something more than you do. This will give you an opportunity to give back, to help people, and to improve someone's life.

You'll find that money is not the only source of happiness and well-being. You will see people who are happy and healthy, not because of money, but because they are engaged in life. They have developed meaning in their lives, and they enjoy positive interaction with people. None of these things are related to having money.

Volunteering can give you inspiration.

Volunteering creates lifelong memories. Work with your high school-aged son or daughter building houses for Habitat for Humanity*. You will be working together as a team of carpenters, sharing meals with community volunteers, becoming friends with people from all over the world, learning new skills, and experiencing the feeling of camaraderie and helping people.

A final thought about volunteering. Getting paid for the work will change the experience. If you get paid there are expectations, even though they may not be explicit. You'll feel the pressure to meet these expectations. You'll be open to criticism. Finally, there is no positive feeling of working with a team because power-based leadership develops. You'll have to continually fight to stay at the top or put up with harassment and degrading insults at the bottom. This turns meaning and enjoyment into stress and resentment.

Volunteer for meaning, enjoyment, and growth.

Give away some of your money. Give money to a person, a community, or a nonprofit project. This is the hardest thing in the world to do. Why? Because you have to work so hard to make money and you enjoy spending the money the way you want to. We are used to spending the money on something for us, even if buying something for someone else, it's still spending money for something we want to do. Giving away money is painful not only because you lose the opportunity to personally spend the money the way you want, but also the recipient may not spend your money the way you'd like.

An adage notes that if you give away money, eventually you will receive more in return. This is rare. More commonly, you will not receive money in return, but you will receive two subtle but important lessons.

Humility. Being humble is being outside of yourself. You are not in control. You are blindly trusting someone or an organization to use the money in a beneficial way.

Responsibility. Giving money away makes you a more responsible person because you will have to live well with the money you have left over.

Giving away money is buying meaning to life.

Other reasons to give away money? People who give money away find it rewarding. Studies have shown giving away money makes people happy. People giving money to others feel more happiness than people spending money on themselves. Give a group of college students $20 and ask half of them to buy something for themselves and the other half to buy something for someone else. The second group scores higher on the happiness scale. Giving money to others brings happiness.

An unusual reason to give money away is that it makes a person feel wealthier. People feel more satisfied with life when they feel wealthier.

Find a purpose in life. Purpose in life is bigger than yourself. You need to know what your purpose in life is. It doesn't require a complex journey or series of questions. It is not complicated. Keep it simple. You only want to know the single, underlying general purpose. There are only a few of these. Specifics come later.

How do you know what your purpose is? Ask yourself the question. You will have the answer. These include *you want to help people, you want to improve people's lives,* or *you want to bring joy to people's lives.* One of these will provide a lifelong anchor to refer back to as you move forward.

This anchor comes to life when you explore specific action on a day-to-day basis. Explore one step further. You want to help people who are poor. You want to improve people's lives by building a business. You want to bring joy to children.

Explore another level. You want to help people who are poor in the Appalachian Mountains. You want to improve people's lives by building a health business. You want to bring joy to children in a hospital.

Now, another level, how are you going to fulfill this purpose? You want to help people who are poor in the Appalachian Mountains by doing a volunteer project. You want to improve people's lives by building a health business with a product for self-healing. You want to bring joy to children in a hospital by bringing an upbeat gift.

Another level, what is today's action step? You want to help people who are poor in the Appalachian Mountains by doing a volunteer project and applying for the project within the next 48 hours. You want to improve people's lives by building a health business with a product for self-healing and building a prototype within 30 days. You want to bring joy to children in a hospital by bringing an upbeat gift within the next ten days.

Your basic purpose remains constant, yet this drilling down system provides you with your lifetime work. The possibilities are endless. You can change the details daily, monthly, or yearly. You can work for a company or start your own company that helps people, that improves people's lives, or that brings joy to people.

There are many benefits of living your life based on your fundamental purpose. You are in charge of your life. You can be yourself. Your activity is enjoyable, and it doesn't feel like work. You are good at it because you are using your natural talents. You are a unique person and will bring your unique approach. Importantly, you will be free of stress, no reason for blame, excuses, complaining, or criticism. You will have a creative and enjoyable life.

Create energy from your job. Does your job take all the energy you have? You can turn work into meaning and energy. Some people are able to do this naturally. For most, however, it's a learned response. The good news is that almost everyone, no matter what their job is, can learn to create positive energy while working.

How is it possible to gain energy from a job? You walk into the office or store or factory, and you're instantly faced with people who start using up your energy. Your boss has extra work for you and throws in a negative comment about last week's project. Your first sale involves somebody complaining about the product, or worse, complaining about you. Your supervisor gives you a team of workers who are lazy. This all occurs in the first 15 minutes after you arrive, and the day continues on the same path for the next eight to ten hours. All of these situations require your energy, and there's nothing left at the end of the day for you or for your family.

A Stanford professor asked an eager group of medical students during the first day of class, "Do you want to be a gas-tank doctor or a solar-panel doctor? Confused, the students asked what he was talking about.

Your first patient in the morning has high blood pressure and a new problem. The next patient has diabetes, high blood pressure, and heart failure requiring additional diagnostic thinking and testing. The third patient brings the family into your office and is confused about medication. The patients continue, one after another, each with more complicated issues. You help each one, providing excellent care – using the energy required to think about each problem, develop a plan, and maintain a positive attitude – but by noon your energy gas tank is less than half full, and you have the entire afternoon to see patients. By the time you return home, the tank is empty. You want to enjoy seeing your family and getting away from work, but you have no energy to do anything but complain and feel miserable. This is a gas-tank doctor.

Let's look at another approach. You see your first patient, and about halfway through you are feeling warmth and compassion toward the patient and for yourself as you realize you're grateful that you have developed the skill and training to help this person. The feeling of gratitude and compassion propels you throughout the day and you return home with renewed energy to spend time with your family or doing any other enjoyable activity. This is a solar-panel doctor.

Ask yourself, while at work, are you a gas-tank person or a solar-panel person?

It's possible to gain energy during the workday. The best way is to start with a huge amount of energy from your required amount of sleep, exercise, and healthy nutrition. Concentrate on positive events. Shrug off negative comments and events, let them pass through you without using energy to judge them or fight them. Finally, gain energy through positive interactions with people and focus on successes, no matter how small.

Create energy by doing work that's aligned with your character and your passion. If you are doing work you love and you're passionate about, three things happen. First, it's not work and you enjoy it. Second, you're good at it. And, third, there's no real competition because your work is unique, and no one else has the same approach that you do.

Make an effort to find your talents and skills. Use this definition of talent – it's your recurrent activities that you enjoy doing every day. You randomly find yourself thinking about these activities in your mind. You keep thinking about them year after year. You have about three to five among the more than 30 identifiable specific talents. Learn what they are. They're your strengths. Create your work environment to use them, and you'll find more meaning and enjoyment in your day.

For example, if you have a passion for numbers, balancing the books can be the biggest thrill of the day for you. This is a talent. That's what you should do because the work will be non-stressful and easy to do. Balancing the numbers will produce positive energy. Your personality aligned with your work brings meaning to your life.

If you have a talent and a passion for music or art, learn how to create a work situation that will allow you to do this all day and provide a source of income. Turning this into reality is no small task, and becoming an entrepreneur in whatever way it takes to translate your vision into actuality is a huge endeavor. However, there are teachers, mentors, programs, and unlimited resources that can assist in this process. The reward in terms of energy and enjoyment is worth the expended effort.

Do you have a job doing the same routine day in and day out to make money so you can do what you love to do after work hours? Don't let it take all of your energy. Use your talent strengths. Find a new way of doing things. Volunteer for extra work. Help someone. Start early. Stay late. Three things will happen. The job will be more enjoyable. You're more likely to be given a promotion and a raise. And, you'll increase your energy so much that you'll go beyond this job and obtain a new job that you love and pays twice as much.

Marcia had an entry-level job of double-checking numbers on the computer for a financial company, potentially extremely tedious and boring. However, she had taken an internet-based, self-analytical series of questions to determine her specific talents. She found that she was highly capable of three-dimensional thinking, and one of her talents was referred to as analytical. She applied these findings to her job. She developed an intricately interconnected spreadsheet program that decreased the time for preparing quarterly reports from three days to three hours. This was such a huge advance that her salary was doubled, and her software program opened the potential for a royalty-based income stream.

Look for the good things at work, engage in positive interactions with people, help others, and let the negative events at the workplace pass through you without a loss of energy. Find and create work that will utilize your talents. Your passion for the work will energize your life.

There are three ways to approach work.

First approach, it's a job. You apply for work to get a job, go through the interviews, accept the job, and work 40 hours a week. It's a job. It brings in money to pay bills and provide life's necessities. You show up to work on time, do the job with no complaints and no resentment, go home and enjoy time away from work. It's part of your life, like brushing teeth. This can be successful for some people whose work is equal to their skills, and they're able to maintain a positive attitude; however, this is rare.

Second approach, it's a career. You do the entry-level job that's boring and not challenging, but you know you will get to the next step soon. You work hard to get to the next step. However, during this process, you find yourself complaining and being critical of others. This may go on for several years, but you eventually obtain the next level and begin working toward the next rung on the ladder. The complaints become more consistent because the work is harder and now you're competing with others, resulting in stress and blame. It's a career and if you keep working, you will eventually be rewarded with a prestigious title and large amount of money. Yet, what will be the state of your mental health? And more importantly, what will the effects be of not really enjoying life during the 20- to 30-year process?

Third approach, it's a calling. Your work is based on something bigger than you. There are three phases to this process. The experimenting phase begins in your teens and 20s with trying new opportunities. It begins with an interest in something and doing this repeatedly until it becomes enjoyable or until you try another interest.

Eventually you stay with something. Then comes the second phase of hours, days and years of practice. This is not passive and mindless practice. This is referred to as "deliberate" practice which has three components: continuous learning everything you can about the craft, creating a defined purpose for each practice, and developing an immediate feedback system to measure improvement. In addition, each deliberate practice session is designed to advance a specific part of the new skill.

The third phase of your life's purpose and calling is doing this day in and day out without effort, no thought of doing anything else, and having a profound impact on people's lives and the community. Sometimes, you will experience the thrill of flow, which has been discussed – the feeling of everything going smoothly, nothing goes wrong, being at the top of your game, and not wanting to stop.

What's for you – a job, a career, or a calling? Explore your life, see where you are, and determine where you want to go. Doing what you like to do (with an occasional bump), every day, all the time, is a wonderful life.

"It's all about me" is an important part of life as we need to take care of ourselves before helping others.

But, in a social setting, "it's always about the other person."

Kindness comes from the heart. Be kind. When you're driving – don't tailgate and let the other person make a left turn. When you're shopping, be kind to the salespeople and to other shoppers. When you're in a restaurant, be kind to the staff and to other people eating. When you're at work, be kind to everyone – work will be more pleasant and productive.

CHAPTER 5
ACCOMPLISHMENTS
PROPEL YOU TO
WELL-BEING

Accomplishments are the fourth component of well-being. They can be major long-term achievements or smaller short-term accomplishments. Doing your daily chores makes you feel good and gives you a warm feeling of well-being throughout the day. Think of these "to-do" tasks as completing one page of a report or one step of a project. Each accomplishment creates positive feelings that form the basis of well-being.

Procrastination is the enemy of accomplishment. Use the ten-second rule. Do something to get going for at least ten seconds. Do anything. A tiny step. Clean the house? Put your hand on the vacuum cleaner. Write a report? Click out a single word. Call your next sale? Tap the name on your contact list. Once you do this, you continue, then you find yourself so engrossed in the activity that you have forgotten about your idle time and complete the task.

Keep your positive brain regions healthy to experience the benefits of accomplishments. We have several realms in our brains that want to dominate and direct our day-to-day actions. All of them want to be in complete control at all times. There are regions that promote positive aspects to our lives, but you need adequate sleep, exercise, and good nutrition to keep them healthy. There are regions that can lead us to bad decisions, anger, addictions, and day and night partying. They thrive on no sleep, no exercise, and junk food.

The single best region is the prefrontal cortex. It's the most powerful and fundamental region of the brain that makes us human. This region is the judgment region, where we make decisions that are best for us and that help us lead a successful day-to-day life. While this is the most powerful region of the brain, it's also the most sensitive to outside forces. Insufficient sleep, lack of exercise, poor-quality food, and not meditating take this region offline and render it nonfunctional.

The other useful realm for accomplishment is the creative region that connects the right and left brain hemispheres, referred to as the *corpus callosum*. This region too requires a healthy lifestyle for peak functioning. Surprisingly, in order for this region to dominate, the prefrontal lobe must be taken offline. This is seen in children who have not yet fully developed their prefrontal lobe, which allows them to daydream and be creative without guilt or stress. The dangers of taking the frontal lobe offline by hormones, alcohol, or drugs can be seen in the outcomes of bad decisions made by children entering their teenage years and by people in their early 20s. After age 25, meditation is an effective way to safely quiet the prefrontal lobe and allow for active creative thinking.

The third positive realm is the hypothalamus, a small region in the limbic system shaped like a hippopotamus that takes care of the minute-by-minute memory system involving people, places, and events. Keep this region in good working order with adequate sleep, exercise, and healthy nutrition.

Now to the schemers. The first is the most dangerous region in the brain, the amygdala. It's the anger center. This region can take control of your actions for hours, days, and even years. It's the center where your thoughts of anger originate. The thoughts can turn to rage with increased heart rate, increased blood pressure, flushed face, and stronger muscle power leading to violence. These thoughts can turn to depression with feelings of isolation and thoughts of dread. The thoughts can recur and lead to chronic anger toward people, governments, places, ideas, and even yourself. Intentions of achieving positive accomplishments are abandoned.

Unlike the prefrontal cortex, the amygdala is an ancient, primitive region of the brain that requires no sleep and thrives on junk food and no exercise. The amygdala can take the prefrontal cortex offline and control all day-to-day actions when you're not getting enough sleep, not exercising, making poor food choices, and when you are ill.

A seemingly less dangerous region is the nucleus accumbens, the pleasure center. This can be a desirable and useful brain center when it's used for positive conditioning when learning new healthy behaviors such as eating healthy foods or breaking bad and dangerous habits. When used at the subconscious level for positive reinforcement, this center can act as a feedback loop with the decision-making prefrontal cortex reinforcing healthy habits.

However, this region can take control of your actions in a bad way, usually just for a matter of hours but sometimes for weeks, and in rare situations, for years. It can be the addiction center, and the endless, out-of-control party center. The feeling you have at a party originates in this region and the pleasurable effects from alcohol or drugs comes from this center, resulting in the addictive nature of these substances as well as the addictive nature of wanting to return to any event that brings pleasure. As with the amygdala, this is a primitive ancient region of emotions that in a bad way can function with no sleep, no exercise, or illness. For bad behaviors, this center will dismantle the good decision-making prefrontal cortex.

The dorsal striatum of the basal ganglia is a small region near the accumbens and a close cousin that causes bad habits like eating too much, napping all day, watching video clips, and checking emails every few minutes. Keep this region in check by keeping a healthy frontal cortex.

You will achieve accomplishments faster and more frequently when your prefrontal cortex is functioning at peak levels by getting sufficient sleep, making healthy food choices, exercising, and meditating. Accomplishments result in self-confidence, a positive outlook for the future, and the feeling of well-being.

CHAPTER 6
SUSTAINABLE POSITIVE
SOCIAL INTERACTION

Positive social interaction is the final component of well-being and can be a powerful self-sustaining trait.

Positive daily interaction with people is healthy for all participants. Talking to coworkers, clerks, shop owners, and restaurant staff in a positive way increases personal energy and feeling good.

Visualize two people talking – spouses, friends, or coworkers. One of them is excited about a huge event and can't wait to tell the other person. The other person has four options. The best option is to respond with engagement and enthusiasm and to ask questions about when, where, and who is involved. A second type of response is a passive "that's nice," not harmful, but a missed opportunity for both people to experience positive feelings from the interaction.

Two options are harmful. The third type of response is to ignore the person's excitement and one-up the conversation with a better or more exciting event. You may have been at a dinner party, work party, or family holiday get-together and noticed certain people having these types of interactions during the entire gathering. This is not an uplifting, pleasant social interaction.

The fourth option is responding with a destructive comment, which happens too often between husbands and wives and between coworkers. It goes like this. Someone can't wait to see the other person to tell them about an exciting event, and is hit with a negative response such as "While you were having fun, I was stressed out trying to work" or "How much is this going to cost us?" Caustic, angry responses destroy the person's story and make the person feel terrible. This type of response is usually triggered because the other person is in a bad mood or angry and lashes out at the first available person.

Use the first response for the best results. It helps both people. The first person gets to feel good again about sharing an exciting event and the second person feels good because of sharing an exciting experience. Eliminate one-up and destructive responses. There is no place for them in positive social interaction.

Positive social interaction: the successful survivor is the person who is starving and gives the last piece of food to someone else. The successful team member is the person who is physically and mentally exhausted with nothing left and extends a hand to help another team member.

There is a dark side of social interaction. In addition to destructive, caustic, one-up social communication, there's another dark side. It's called the toxic "dark triad" personality. People with the dark triad personality are dangerous to your health. They could be your friend, boss, supervisor, or coworker.

The psychological terms used for the triad are *narcissism, Machiavellianism,* and *psychopathy.*

We know narcissism as self-centeredness and egocentricity, but in the context of social interaction, extreme narcissism is the total disregard for other people's feelings. This is especially hurtful in the workplace where the boss loudly berates an employee for a minor mistake with anger and meanness in the voice. The employee already knows about the mistake and will never repeat it again. This painful public humiliation is likely to linger for weeks or months and makes the workplace stressful and depressing for the entire staff. Ultimately, this fear-based leadership will destroy the organization or company. Alternatively, positive social interaction with employees helps everyone feel better and be more productive.

Machiavellianism is a more subtle trait to recognize because as a friend, coworker, or employee, you don't know what evil action is going on. Dark-triad people will do anything to benefit themselves by exploiting and manipulating others. These people have their own agenda and any help or favor they ask of you is for their own gain, and almost always at a huge cost to you, which you don't know about. This can take the form of covering up a seemingly innocent event at work or providing a fabricated excuse. Requests made by ruthless people lead to trouble. Honest and non-deceptive social interactions eliminate such threats.

Psychopathy is medically abnormal. It's the psychopath personality. In the extreme, it leads to mass murders. The psychopathy component of the dark triad has its basis in impulsive, unpredictable social actions. Individuals with this personality are callous, showing a satisfied smirk when delivering bad news or criticizing a friend or employee. The worse trait for psychopathy is the feeling of having no remorse, a characteristic that likely developed as a neglected infant or child. Positive social interaction involves none of these feelings.

Let's return to positive social interaction, no judgment. One aspect of positive social interaction is not judging people. Walk into a room filled with people, look around, and have no judgment. No one has faults. They are who they are without your feelings about who they should be. This makes you feel good. Judging people means you are comparing yourself to others for validation of who you are. Being nonjudgmental frees the need for comparison, resulting in increased personal energy and sense of well-being.

Bring out the best in people. Do you know people who can instantly charge your battery and give you positive energy? Being near them, talking to them, and interacting with them energizes you. Stay with them. They're good for your health. Better yet, become one of these people yourself and spread the energy.

Hans and Nell are a depressing couple. Ask Hans how he's doing, and he'll say, "Not bad for a dead man." He finds something negative to say about everything. Nell is the same way. She always has a negative comment. Ask her about attending a celebration, and she'll say it's no fun because there are too many people. A holiday trip turns into one complaint after another – the flight is delayed, the food is bad, the taxi is too expensive, the room isn't ready, it's too hot, it's too cold, it's too sunny, or it's raining. Her mind is filled with so many negative thoughts and complaints, she misses the beautiful scenery and interesting people around her. And if the couple enters a room together, they drain the energy from everyone around them.

Not so with Coe and Jill. Coe always has an upbeat hello for everyone, and he makes people feel special. He doesn't dwell on the negative things about people or ideas. Jill has a sparkling personality. She smiles all the time. She has a special ability to find something positive about everyone she sees during the day. She compliments salespeople on their friendly service or their smile or their clothing. She talks to people at restaurants as if they were lifelong friends. She's not afraid to engage kids – she draws them out and finds out what they like, making them feel special. When Coe and Jill enter a room, they fill it with energy for everyone around them.

You may not want to be as extreme as Coe and Jill, but their basic approach to life is positive, enjoyable, and worthy of emulation.

The science behind the transfer of positive energy between people is related to the creation of "feel-good" neurotransmitters. These include phenylethylamine, or PEA, which increases the activity of other neurotransmitters such as dopamine, which gives the feeling of pleasure; norepinephrine, which is a stimulator; acetylcholine, for improved mental activity; and especially serotonin, which can regulate impulse control, preventing hostile interaction. PEA is highly concentrated in the limbic system, or the emotional center of the brain, which increases motivation and feelings. Oxytocin is also involved as the bonding hormone neurotransmitter.

Positive community interaction is good for your health and well-being. For example, over 100 years ago, a group of individuals came to the United States from a small village in Italy. They settled in a Pennsylvania location and stayed in the small town for generations. They were similar to people in surrounding villages. They ate the same foods, did the same amount of exercise, and had the same types of jobs. However, no one under the age of 65 had a heart attack from inflamed arteries, but a high percentage of people in the surrounding villages did. Why?

The only difference between the two groups was the amount of community trust. Over many generations, members of this community built a vast amount of trust among themselves. Everyone knew they could count on other community members to help them if they had problems or were in trouble. No one in the community would hurt anyone, and they all forgave each other. Neighbors always tried to help as much as they could.

As a result, the stress level was low compared to that of surrounding towns. People knew they could find help from their community. There was no chronic stress and no cortisol response causing inflammation. There were healthy hearts and increased vitality.

For effective positive social interaction, being kind exceeds being nice. If you think about it, we have been told the virtues of being nice to people since childhood. But, being nice to people may be considered a duty and means trying to please people. Being kind to people comes from the heart and is meaningful interaction. Be kind to people for improved well-being.

Have a job interview? Giving a pitch? Need help with your project? Success is not related to qualifications and experience, this is well-known. Success is related to the likable factor. Be likable, use positive communication. Use compliments. People remember two parts of the interaction: a peak accomplishment or event, and the end of a conversation. So, if you have a weakness, bring it up early, and it will be forgotten. End with a life-changing accomplishment or a world-class feature, and it will be remembered.

Love, the ultimate positive social interaction. Everyone knows that falling in love increases your heart rate. Did you know that increasing your heart rate will help you fall in love with the person next to you? Try it and find out.

Want to fall in love with your husband or wife, your girlfriend or boyfriend, or a first date? Do something that increases your heart rate, especially something requiring cooperation together, like keeping a kayak in a straight line. Go for a hike, climb a mountain, take a ride on a bike path, take ballroom dancing lessons, work out together, or go for a run together.

That's what happened to me. I was training for the New York Marathon along the Charles River in Boston and saw someone, my future wife, Joan, coming my direction and made the U-turn. Our hearts were beating fast. It didn't take long, a few moments, to fall in love.

This is what happens. The feel-good hormones and neurotransmitters like endorphin, serotonin, and dopamine kick in from the exercise, and when two people exercise, the bonding hormone oxytocin is flowing. In addition, with exercise and increased heart rate, both of you are in the alpha-brainwave world of happiness and bliss.

Joan and I ran the Greek Marathon for our first anniversary and our favorite memories were running the three 20-mile training runs to Wellesley and back to Boston the three Saturdays before the marathon. We were together in the alpha-brainwave meditation state, a fantasy world filled with love, joy, and peace. The hot-fudge sundae at the end was also a big plus.

I was talking with my friend during a Cape Cod ocean swim telling him about increasing the heart rate to fall in love. This reminded him of his first date with his wife – they took ballroom dancing together, just the two of them. Heart rates increased, they fell in love, and were married within the year. My friend John hiked a mountain trail with someone new and fell in love.

Meet in a gym and fall in love.

That's what happened to Gertrude and Alvin, who tied the knot at ages 98 and 94 after having met at the gym and worked out together eight years (*New York Times*). Work out together, increase the heartbeats, and fall in love.

There's a bonus. You will create lifelong memories that you will both recall ten years later, 20 years later, and forever. Remember nighttime skating on the Brookline Country Club pond, remember the New Hampshire hike with cranberry nut bread and Mozart's music, remember running by MIT during a Boston wintery nor'easter, and remember the hike to the top of Angel Mountain in the San Francisco Bay with the beautiful changes in trees, shrubs, and flowers with each change of elevation.

Want to enjoy life together? First date? Do things together that will you increase both of your heart rates. Run together, stay together. Love is in the air.

CHAPTER 7
YOU GOTTA LOVE LIFE: THE FIRST OF TEN HEALTH PRACTICES

Life is to be enjoyed. Adopt the attitude that it's going to be a great day filled with new experiences, meeting new people, and seeing friends. Start the day with gratitude for the opportunity to have an exciting day. Start the morning with anticipation and the simple expectation: "This is going to be a great day!"

Let me tell you about my friend and work-out partner John. At age 50, which was 15 years ago, he developed a vague discomfort in his belly that wouldn't go away. After long and extensive probing, a cancer in his left kidney was discovered. In a matter of hours, the cancer along with the kidney was surgically chopped out. John returned to his life of enjoying every day and forgot about the cancer, erasing it from his mind.

In addition to being joyful, John is a grateful person. He is grateful for everything, his surgeons, his medical team, his hospital, his family, his friends, and his work. This may be his natural personality, but it may have developed during his teenage years when he was an automobile mechanic and living in an abandoned car in a country far away from the United States. He knew it was a temporary situation, and he was always on the lookout for an opportunity to better his life. The chance presented itself when his uncle helped him come to America, where he learned to be an expert mechanic.

The next opportunity John seized was finding a way to purchase abandoned gas stations from large American corporations. This led to multiple purchases and over the years he built a successful enterprise. John was able to provide for his family and for his extended family across the ocean – paying back the help that he received from his uncle. During this whole time, John loved life. He loved the big picture and he loved the details. He loved his work and especially loved being with his family and friends.

Suddenly, six years after removal of the kidney cancer, an unsettling abdominal pain developed and sent him back for diagnostic studies. This time, the answer was worse – pancreas cancer, a six-month killer that has prematurely ended the lives of so many people, including founders of billion-dollar companies, actors, comedians, and political leaders. But not John, he chose surgery that successfully removed the entire cancer without difficulty. But the next day a series of complications began that kept John in the intensive care unit for 40 days. He recalled waking from the ordeal and being so weak that he was not able to lift his arm to eat.

Fortunately, John took the advice of his doctor, who told him to exercise his way back to health. John loved life and wanted to live on his terms, and if exercise was going to make that a reality, he was going to exercise. And exercise he did: 5:30 a.m. body pump, 6:30 to 7:30 walking around the indoor track with his friends, and 7:30 to 8:30 spin class. This was his daily routine for several years.

However, this routine was interrupted two years ago with an ominous chest X-ray finding. There were spots in John's lungs that were slowly growing in size. They were from tumors that had spread from that kidney cancer so many years ago.

John had a decision to make: continue observation until his lungs filled with tumors or choose surgery to have them removed. He believed in "getting on with living" not "getting on with dying." He chose life despite the one-in-five chance of dying on the table from the operation. He wasn't going to wait two to three years for death.

The highly skilled surgeons removed 22 tumors from John's lungs, and the technological advances at this world-class hospital helped him through the first day. But, he developed complications from pneumonia the next day that gave him a 1-in-a-100 chance of surviving. Three days later, his remaining kidney failed, forcing him to dialysis and a 1-in-a-1,000 chance of surviving. A few days later, a massive heart attack left him on the extracorporeal membrane oxygenation (ECMO) machine with a 1-in-10,000 chance of surviving, which was soon followed by a stroke, decreasing his odds of survival to 1-in-100,000. At day 30 in the intensive care unit, he developed blood clots that gave him a one-in-a-million chance of survival.

John survived this ordeal and continues to work out with me every day. How did he outlast all odds? He had phenomenal surgeons, medical doctors, and support equipment plus hundreds and thousands of prayers, and theta healing. All of these helped, but he survived for one reason. He did his part, he wanted to live. He loved life.

John can't wait for the day to start. He can't wait to see his wife, his daughter, his three sons, he can't wait to see his friends and work out, and he can't wait to go to work. He enjoys every minute of the day and shares his love of life with everyone near him.

This extraordinary person exemplifies the first health practice: love life. John is always engaged in life and an active participant. He's always doing something. He has meaning in life, and he puts his family before everything else. He's happy and grateful for what he has. He's always smiling and has a friendly hello for everyone. He forgives people and gives them as many chances as they need to try again. He always engages in positive social interaction. It's not about him – it's always about the other person. How's everyone else doing? He doesn't dwell on past difficulties. He doesn't complain, blame, criticize, or make excuses. John exercises every day at the workout facility for at least one hour and often longer with a few breaks for talking and spreading good cheer among his friends. John knows who he is and enjoys the freedom this allows him.

Joseph Campbell in *The Power of Myth* explains that myths do not portray searching for the meaning of life, but rather that the meaning of life is actually the experience of living life. It's the experience of being alive that counts. That's why the stories about Greek gods have persisted forever – they're about extreme emotions of fear, greed, death, and love. People need to experience emotions to feel alive.

Look to the future as time to enjoy, be productive, learn something new, and have positive interactions with intriguing people. Look for the good in all things. Free your mind to do what you wish. That's loving life.

CHAPTER 8
NUTRITION IS A
LIFESTYLE, NOT A DIET

A healthy nutrition lifestyle means eating the right food, in the right amount, at the right time, and preparing the food in a healthy manner.

More than 90 percent of the food we eat can be harmful. These foods have added sugar, added salt, too much saturated fat, and too much processed omega-6 fat. There's not enough omega-3 fat and not enough fiber. Harmful foods cause inflammation throughout the body and the arteries, resulting in heart disease, diabetes, hypertension, stroke, and cancer.

Without our knowledge, the vast majority of foods include multi-ingredient processed foods with added sugar, added salt, and processed omega-6 fats. Many are sweet and sugar-based foods and beverages, salty foods, and saturated-fat fried foods.

Ultra-processed foods include breads, cereals, salty snacks, sweets, and sodas. These processed foods are making people overfed and undernourished because they are high in added sugars and low in nutrients. Sugar is hiding in all sorts of packaged foods, and these processed foods account for almost all of the added sugars in American diets.

For example, go to your nearby convenience store and see that there are no beverages available among the hundreds of items in the refrigerated units that are safe in the quantities offered. They have too much sugar, too much salt, or both. Look at the snacks, pastries, chips, and even the "healthy" energy bars and find excessive amounts of saturated fats, processed omega-6 fats, sugar, and sodium.

People often wonder why we are told that a certain food is healthy today and a year later, we're told the same food is not healthy. This is because human nutrition is complex and requires long-term research to find answers. That's why it's important to continually learn about nutrition as it will change in the future, and that's why it's important to base your food choices on documented research and not conditioned public responses.

Another reason why nutrition is complicated is because metabolism varies from person to person as everyone has a unique genetic makeup.

Nutrition is dose-related. Some foods are beneficial in small amounts but deadly in high amounts. The interaction between two or more foods is complex, sometimes resulting in safe foods, but sometimes resulting in harmful foods.

Finally, although cell-culture testing is helpful for major life-threatening effects, multicultural population studies are required to confirm healthy foods, and these are expensive and take a minimum of ten years.

For all of these reasons and more, we don't have all the answers, yet we have made large advances in finding healthy, non-harmful nutrition. Everyone should try to keep up with the latest information, and apply recommendations for a longer, disease-free life.

Misleading information about foods is a major issue that requires caution when learning about nutrition. Keep in mind that the number of viewers and internet clicks determines the viability of media outlets and websites, so titles of news stories or articles are written to attract viewers and clicks.

For example, a website title states: "Lima Beans Are Poison" or "Rhubarb Will Kill You." The purpose of these titles is to get more hits on the site. Yet, most people only read and remember the titles. And these titles can be harmful because people will stop eating lima beans and rhubarb, yet these two foods are healthy if prepared in the right way, eaten in the right amount, and at the right time.

Most people glance at the title and move onto another topic yet the thought is registered in the subconscious mind and lima beans are taken off the food list. The text goes on to say that lima beans contain the poison arsenic; however, this can be said of almost all foods, medicines, and water.

Arsenic naturally occurs in soil and water throughout the world and may occur at the molecular level in almost all foods. It's a dose-related issue – a small amount does nothing and too much kills people. That's why food, pharmaceutical, and beverage companies continually test their products for unacceptable levels of arsenic before selling them to consumers.

Lima beans are on the list of healthy foods. They are not harmful as implied by the title. They have no cholesterol and are low in saturated fat. They're also a good source of protein, folic acid, iron, potassium, manganese, and fiber.

What about rhubarb, will it kill you? It's the rhubarb leaves that can be harmful, and then only if eaten in large amounts. It's like not eating cherry pits or peach seeds. Rhubarb leaves are not sold at the market, and people that grow their own rhubarb know that the leaves are not to be eaten. The title of the website text is once again misleading and results in the loss of a healthy food source. Rhubarb has a low glycemic index, no saturated fat, and no cholesterol, plus it's a good source of vitamin C, vitamin K, calcium, potassium, manganese, and fiber.

These two examples illustrate the power of certain emotional words in website titles and articles. When we find something that may be useful, we want to spread the word to our friends and family. Sometimes this can save lives, but sometimes it can be harmful, and become a conditioned response without factual basis.

For example, you may have heard that vaccines cause autism. This is false and based on a single fraudulent report in a February 1998 prestigious medical journal. Look up the report, it says "retracted" in big red letters across every page of the article. The person who wrote the article falsified the numbers for his own personal benefit at the expense of his colleagues and the public. He was severely punished for his actions.

There was no basis for his statement, yet millions of people spread the word and parents stopped having their children vaccinated, governments launched investigation committees into the vaccine industry, and some unvaccinated children died. The word was spread because the headline and article used fear. Few people spread the word about the fraud because it was too bland for people to share. This is a dramatic example of how false information can spread by word-of-mouth from a single fraudulent source.

There are two major lessons from this example. First, be aware of emotional words that are used in titles to get you to view the article. If people want views, they use emotional words that drive action.

Emotional words on the positive list include *joy, happiness,* and *excitement;* negative words include *anger, frustration,* and *fear.* These words provoke action and clicks. Words that don't get clicks include *sad, confusion, shame, guilt, contentment,* and *satisfaction.*

Spreading the word about healthy nutrition can be helpful; however, make sure the information is evidence-based and if necessary read the original article.

What are harmful foods and what makes them harmful? Harmful foods contain added sugar, added salt, too much processed omega-6 fats, too much saturated fats, and contain manufactured trans-fats. These substances cause high triglyceride (trigs) and low-density lipoprotein (HDL) levels in the blood directly cause inflammation of the interior walls of the arterial blood vessels.

What's sucrose sugar? It's table sugar and comes from sugarcane or sugar beets. Whether the sugar is from an organic source or non-organic source, it's still sugar. The chemical structure is a combination of two simple sugars – glucose and fructose.

Glucose is the sugar measured in the blood and the sugar that increases to dangerous levels in individuals with diabetes.

Fructose is the *naturally occurring sugar* found in fruit and is not harmful in small amounts. High-fructose corn syrup is a *manufactured sweetener.* Sucrose and high-fructose corn syrup are the sugars added to unhealthy supermarket drinks and foods, sometimes in huge quantities making them harmful.

Added sugar is a problem because it causes inflammation throughout the body, which results in inflammation-based diseases, including heart disease, stroke, diabetes, metabolic syndrome, hypertension, and cancer. In addition, sugar also causes inflammatory-based immune dysfunction diseases.

Eating too much sugar increases your blood sugar level, which in turn produces an insulin spike. Insulin is a hormone made by the pancreas and binds to the blood sugar and takes this glucose into the cell for energy.

Too much insulin and too many insulin spikes lead to insulin resistance, which causes diabetes and inflammation of the arteries.

Insulin no longer functions properly and can't remove glucose from the blood causing increased blood glucose levels. In addition, this dysfunctional insulin can't remove triglycerides from the blood causing increased levels of these stored fats. The high triglyceride levels in the blood cause direct inflammation of the thin internal walls of the arteries, leading to stiff, narrow arteries resulting in heart attacks and strokes.

Sugar causes visceral adipose tissue, or belly fat, which is intra-abdominal fat close to intestinal organs. Visceral adipose tissue is also fat stored around other visceral organs such as the heart, liver, kidney, and pancreas. Unlike adipose tissue or fat below the skin on the upper arms or legs, visceral belly fat is inflammation.

How does added sugar cause fat bellies? Sugar causes resistance to the hormone leptin, the body's hormone that tells you to stop eating. Leptin is secreted by fat cells. As fat cells fill up with fat, leptin is released and shuts down the urge to eat more. This takes time, usually about 20 minutes, which is a good reason to eat slowly. The high level of triglycerides from too much sugar blocks leptin from reaching the brain, and with the brain no longer receiving the signal to stop eating, people continue to eat and eat out of control.

In addition to disrupting the function of leptin, the belly fat cells become so stuffed that the cell walls malfunction releasing inflammatory molecules that circulate in the blood, causing inflammatory-based chronic diseases.

A final issue with sugar is that it's addictive. Sugar stimulates the nucleus accumbens reward center of the brain and pleasure receptors producing addictive neurotransmitters. This leads people to crave sugar to experience these feel-good neurotransmitters over and over, always wanting more.

To sum up, why is added sugar so bad for you? It causes insulin resistance, leptin resistance, increased triglyceride fat in the blood, and increased inflamed belly fat, all of which result in heart attacks, hypertension, stroke, diabetes, cancer, and other deadly inflammatory-based diseases.

What's fructose sugar? This is one of the simple sugars that makes up sucrose. In small naturally-occurring amounts, it's good. In high added and concentrated amounts, fructose causes inflammation and increased visceral belly fat just like sucrose sugar.

Fructose is metabolized by the liver and, unlike glucose, does not require insulin. Fructose is in fruit and fruit is healthy in small amounts. But, it's not the fructose that renders fruit healthy, it's the vitamins and, most importantly, the fiber – which acts as a toxic vacuum cleaner. Fruit also has sucrose sugar and some in high amounts, a reason to limit fruit intake, especially fruit juices to four ounces.

High-fructose corn syrup is different from naturally-occurring fructose. It's a manufactured chemical to increase fructose content. The issue with foods and beverages containing large amounts of high-fructose corn syrup is that it's easy to consume too much fructose, which easily overwhelms the liver fructose metabolism system. Read labels – high-fructose corn syrup is everywhere, including in many beverages, cereals, candy bars, cookies and cakes, ice cream, sauces, snacks, and even processed meats.

What's sodium salt? It's table salt and added to foods in the form of sodium chloride. For thousands of years salt was used as a food preservative, but it gradually began to be used to improve the taste of foods. People have become conditioned to the taste of salt, and now it's used everywhere. We need about 1,500 milligrams of sodium daily, which naturally occurs in vegetables and grains. This is the reason added salt is not needed, and if you read the labels on store beverages, you'll see that some of them have 1,500 milligrams in a single small container.

Too much sodium is a problem because studies of thousands of individuals have shown that the amount of a person's salt intake is *directly related* to their risk of heart disease, hypertension, and strokes. *The more salt, the more disease.*

Sugar, fat, and salt foods have become irresistible, to the point of being addicting. Try eating one potato chip, one tiny piece of candy, or one salted peanut. You can't eat just one of these. Try eating a small portion of a box of processed rice with buttery salted chicken or beef flavor, or even a box of quinoa with added salt and fatty chicken broth. You don't eat a small amount of sugar, fat, or salty foods. You eat and eat them until you're Thanksgiving-stuffed, resulting in a bloated stomach and body distress. Most of us have been conditioned to associate these foods with feeling good because we were rewarded with them as special treats throughout childhood. Condition yourself to eat foods with no added sugar and no added salt.

What are processed omega-6 fats? These fats are monounsaturated fats. The number 6 is the location of the unfilled double carbon bond slot on the long-string fatty acid chain making up the unsaturated fats. Omega-6 fat is an essential fatty acid, which means the body does not produce this, and it must be consumed from an outside source. A reasonable amount of omega-6 that occurs naturally in foods is generally not harmful; however, omega-6 is found in processed foods and oils, farmed-raised salmon and fish, caged chickens, and penned-in, corn-fed beef. Too much of this "processed" omega-6 is harmful.

Too much processed omega-6 is a problem because it causes inflammation throughout the body and especially in the internal lining of the arteries, leading to heart attack or stroke. People who have replaced saturated fats with processed omega-6 have increased their risk of heart disease.

Omega-6 was not a problem before the 1950s in the United States and is not currently a problem in many non-industrialized countries. Why? The biggest source of omega-6 today is from processed foods and meats from corn-fed, penned-in beef, caged chickens, and farm-raised fish. The manufacturing technique for food preservation was not available years ago. Free-range animals and free-swimming fish were the norm. In the past, naturally occurring foods resulted in a mostly healthy balance of the inflammation omega-6 and the anti-inflammation omega-3.

Sources of omega-6 are everywhere. Far too many foods that contain too much processed omega-6 are readily available. They are also cheap and taste good. Examples include processed foods, unhealthy deli meats, and vegetable oils such as sunflower oil, corn oil, peanut oil, and soybean oil.

It's paradoxical that in the 1960s corn oil and peanut oil were recommended as a replacement for lard and butter for frying foods because corn oil and peanut oil contained unsaturated fats. Today, after determining that their omega-6 levels were too high, these oils are considered harmful.

Soybeans have a worse story: often thought of as a healthy alternative in the past, today processed oil from soybeans is a big source of omega-6 in the diet throughout the world. Processed soybean oil is in chips, pastries, snacks, ice cream, and fast food.

Processed corn and soy are used for animal feed and farmed-raised fish feed, resulting in a high omega-6 content of these foods.

Meats containing processed omega-6 are common in the US. I recently drove across the country with my family from shining sea to shining sea with purple mountains. In the middle of the country, we experienced a foul-smelling stench for several miles that permeated the car, causing all of us to become nauseous.

There were hundreds and thousands of cattle squeezed tightly in pens next to each other. Were they receiving processed corn and soy feed plus steroid hormones for muscle growth? Probably. These are deplorable conditions, and the meat from these animals would have excessive amounts of omega-6 that would overwhelm the omega-6/omega-3 balance in people.

The same situation may occur with cage-raised chickens and farm-raised salmon, both having too much processed omega-6 fat.

What are saturated fats? These are a long chain of fatty acids with a glycerol backbone and saturated with hydrogen ions, leaving no space for other bonds. Some saturated fats are in the solid white form at room temperature, like lard and the white fat on a steak; others are liquid, like coconut oil and palm oil, and become solid when cold, such as in ice cream.

There are no empty spots for oxygen molecules in saturated fats that can oxidize the molecule, making the fat rancid and spoiled. This is good because these fats are stable; however, we need to limit the amount of saturated fats we eat, preferably less than 20 grams per day, which is only one and a half tablespoons.

High amounts of saturated fats can be found in hamburgers, hot dogs, deli meats, french fries, pizza, fried food, candy bars, donuts, ice cream, and pastries.

The names of some of these saturated fats include *butyric acid,* with 4 carbon atoms contained in butter; *lauric acid,* with 12 carbon atoms contained in coconut oil, palm kernel oil, and breast milk; *myristic acid,* with 14 carbon atoms contained in cow's milk and dairy products; *palmitic acid,* with 16 carbon atoms contained in palm oil and meat; and *stearic acid,* with 18 carbon atoms contained in meat and cocoa butter. Some of these specific saturated fats are beneficial in low amounts, yet all of them cause inflammation in high amounts.

Tallow from melting beef fat or chicken fat contains 90 percent saturated fats, and lard from melting pork fat is high in saturated fatty acids. Palm kernel oil is mostly saturated fat.

Too much saturated fat is harmful because in high amounts, saturated fats increase the fat protein in the blood called *low-density lipoprotein* (LDL). High levels of LDL cause direct inflammation of the lining of arteries throughout the body and result in heart attacks and strokes. The largest increases in LDL are caused by saturated fats in fatty meats, such as bacon, sausage, and marbled steak, and fried foods, such as french fries, fried seafood, and donuts.

The problem with these foods is that we can't eat them in small amounts. We can't eat one french fry or one potato chip. We can easily eat a plate full of french fries and a whole bag of potato chips. Limit saturated fats for a healthy lifestyle.

What are trans-fats? These are manufactured unsaturated fats where the empty carbon and hydrogen sites are filled by hydrogenation. Most unsaturated fats are healthy because these empty bonding sites allow for healthy metabolism; however, trans-fats are an exception. They are the most harmful of all fats.

Although these fats may occur naturally in small amounts in some meats and milk products, an industrial process of hydrogenation was developed during the 1950s that resulted in filling up the empty bonds in unsaturated fats. This turned liquid unsaturated fats into solid, which was used to make margarine.

Soon, manufacturers realized that this industrial process of filling up empty bonds could make foods stable and result in a longer shelf life. As a result, trans-fats were found in thousands of foods, including processed foods, deli meats, cakes, cookies, pies, frosting, biscuits, crackers, cream-filled candies, donuts, and fast foods.

Trans-fats are harmful because studies have shown an increased amount of trans-fat intake is directly correlated with an increased coronary artery disease and heart attacks. The more trans-fats in the diet, the higher the risk.

Trans-fats floating in the blood attach to the internal wall of the small arteries giving blood to the heart, which causes inflammation and plaques that eventually block the arteries, cutting off oxygen and nutrients to the heart.

Studies have also shown that high amounts of trans-fats cause obesity, high blood pressure, and diabetes.

Trans-fats are so likely to cause inflamed coronary arteries and other inflammation throughout the body that the use of manufactured trans-fats has been banned.

What are triglycerides? These are stored fatty acids. When you've burned up the amount of fat needed for the day, the body stores the extra fatty acids as triglycerides. These fats float in the blood and are measured as your "trig" level.

During ancient times, stored fat was used as an emergency supply of energy to survive periods of famine, but today with food available everywhere, persistent high blood trigs are too common, and they are harmful.

What causes high trig levels? Added sugar is the major cause of dangerously high levels. Eating too much sugar causes too much insulin. After the body has reached the storage capacity of the glucose in the form of glycogen, the increased insulin causes the liver to convert glucose into fatty acids and triglycerides, which are transported to fat cells. The triglycerides are in the blood on the way to the fat cells.

Sugar, manufactured corn syrup, sugar-based foods and beverages, refined white bread and pasta, and high glycemic carbohydrates like potatoes cause increased triglyceride levels.

Triglycerides are harmful because high levels cause direct damage and injury to the internal wall of the arteries, making them stiff, inflamed and clogged up – resulting in heart attacks and strokes.

Let's talk about healthy foods. As we've discussed, you need to eat nutritious and non-harmful foods prepared in a healthy manner in the right amount and at the right time.

This can be difficult because there are too many harmful food choices available and not enough healthy food choices. The solution is to learn what the healthy foods are, search out and buy healthy foods, replace harmful foods, and learn to acquire a taste for these foods. It takes time, but the more you eat healthy foods, the more you enjoy them.

Healthy foods are simple, non-processed foods and foods without bar codes. They're grown as naturally as possible with personal attention. They're fruits and vegetables grown organically in well-cultivated fields without pesticides. They're from free-range chickens and animals. They're free-swimming fish in rivers, lakes, and oceans. They're non-processed carbohydrates that have not been fructose-condensed by a manufacturing process, and oils that have not been hydrogenated.

The method for consuming high-quality foods is simpler than you'd think. Eat as close to nature and naturally produced food as you can.

Lean proteins. Protein is good, but beware the company it keeps.

Proteins are made up of long strings of 20 amino acids. There are nine essential amino acids that the body cannot make, such as lysine and tryptophan, and 11 nonessential amino acids that the body can make, such as aspartic acid, glutamine, glycine, and tyrosine. Protein can't be stored, so we need daily intake. If the intake is insufficient, muscle and immune system function can be lost.

Some foods, such as milk, eggs, chicken, fish, and quinoa have complete protein, which means these foods contain all 20 amino acids. Incomplete proteins, found in bread, grains, nuts, legumes, and vegetables, lack one or more amino acids, and additional protein is needed. Body protein and enzyme synthesis will stop if one amino acid is missing; therefore, a balance of protein foods is needed.

Plant-based proteins include the ancient grains such as quinoa, millet, amaranth, and teff. Keep in mind that, with the exception of quinoa and teff, most grains don't have all of the essential amino acids. Detailed nutrition information about these foods and other foods can be found on the website Self-Nutrition Data.

Quinoa is a grain grown in Bolivia and naturally gluten free and a complete protein. In a 100-gram serving, which is about one-half cup, the glycemic load is 10; protein, 2.8 grams; fiber, 1.3 grams; sugar, 0.1grams; folate, 42 micrograms; omega-3, 307 milligrams; omega-6, 2977 milligrams; magnesium, 64 milligrams; potassium, 172 milligrams; sodium, 7 milligrams; and manganese, 0.6 milligrams.

Millet is a gluten-free African grain; 100 grams of cooked millet is slightly less than one-half cup and has a glycemic load of 12; protein, 3.5 grams; fiber, 1.3 grams; sugar, 0.1 grams; omega-3, 28 milligrams; omega-6, 480 milligrams; magnesium, 44 milligrams; potassium, 62 milligrams; sodium, 2 milligrams; and manganese, 0.3 milligrams.

Amaranth is considered a gluten-free Aztec food. In 100 grams, which is about one and a quarter cups, the glycemic load is 9; protein, 3.8 grams; fiber, 2.1 grams; sugar, 1.7 grams; folate, 22 micrograms; omega-3, 42 milligrams; omega-6, 2.7 grams; magnesium, 65 milligrams; potassium, 135 milligrams; sodium, 6 milligrams; and manganese, 0.9 milligrams.

Teff is a gluten-free and complete protein Ethiopian grain and can be used to show the difference between uncooked and cooked grains. The glycemic load is higher for uncooked teff at 43 compared to cooked teff at 10. The protein is lower in cooked at 3.9 grams compared to uncooked at 13.3 grams. Additional composition of the uncooked teff includes fiber, 8.0 grams; sugar, 1.7 grams; omega-3, 135 milligrams; omega-6, 936 milligrams; magnesium, 184 milligrams; potassium, 427 milligrams; sodium, 12 milligrams; and manganese, 9.2 milligrams.

These grains can be a good source of protein, low sodium, and fiber, although they may be high in omega-6 compared to omega-3; therefore, pair these with foods that have high omega-3 fats. In addition, pair these grains with legumes to complete the required protein intake of the 20 amino acids. Sprouted whole grains can also be a good source of protein.

Other plant-based proteins include lentils, peas, kidney beans, black beans, pinto beans, fava beans, chickpeas, broccoli, and leafy green vegetables like spinach.

Fish, chicken, and beef can be excellent sources of complete protein, but exercise caution because of the potential for consuming too much dangerous fat. It's important to eliminate all visible fat in these foods because it's visceral fat containing high amounts of saturated fat.

This is where the issue of farm-raised fish and penned-up poultry and beef is so important. No matter where fish may be farm-raised, the enclosed tight conditions and food that is consumed result in large amounts of processed omega-6 fat, which causes inflammation and heart disease. This is also true for chickens penned up in small cages. It is especially true for cows that live in four-feet-by-six-feet stalls and are fed corn and given anabolic steroids. Fish need to be free-swimming. Poultry and cattle need the free range to eliminate processed omega-6 fats.

The good fats. Unsaturated fats are the healthy ones. These are fats that have empty slots between carbon and hydrogen molecules because there are double bonds in some places along the fatty acid molecules. The bonding sites are unsaturated. This means that unsaturated fats, such as olive oil, need to be kept fresh because over time the unsaturated slots become filled by oxidization, changing these healthy unsaturated fats into damaged, broken-down, rancid fats that cause inflammation. Avoid overripe avocados and non-fresh salmon.

Omega-3 fatty acids are a group of several fatty acids classified as essential fatty acids because we need them. The name is derived from the location of the first double bond – three carbons in from the end.

Omega-3 fatty acids are needed for prostaglandins, which are lipid-based substances with many healthy functions, and omega-3 fatty acids have an anti-inflammatory action. They reduce cardiovascular disease by maintaining elasticity and softness of blood vessels. Omega-3 fatty acids are found in cold-water fish and plant oils such as flaxseed.

Healthy omega-6/omega-3 ratio. Omega-6 fatty acids, just like the omega-3 fatty acids, are essential fatty acids. The name derivation is easy. The first double bond occurs at the sixth spot. In appropriate amounts, omega-6 fatty acids are good for the heart and brain, but unlike omega-3 fatty acids, too much can cause inflammation and cardiovascular disease, especially "processed" omega-6 fat.

Omega-3 fat is also an essential fatty acid and must be consumed from an outside source. Omega-3 fat is anti-inflammatory. Omega-3 fats are found in vegetables such as spinach, winter squash, brussels sprouts,

cauliflower, kale, and free-swimming fish such as salmon. Multiple studies have shown that omega-3 fats prevent heart disease and stroke, and
may protect against autoimmune inflammatory diseases.

Food scientists have discovered something important about these
two unsaturated fats. The body needs an equal balance of omega-6 and
omega-3 for optimal health, because a high omega-6/omega-3 ratio causes
inflammation. There was a healthy balance between these two fatty acids
in our food until manufacturing processes and forced-fed animal practices developed over the past 25 years. Now there is an overpowering
imbalance from 15 to as high as 40 times more omega-6 compared to
omega-3 fatty acids, allowing the inflammatory properties of omega-6 to
damage the lining of the heart and brain arteries, which we know causes
heart attacks and strokes as well as inflammatory responses throughout
the body. Restore the omega-6/omega-3 balance by not eating processed
omega-6 fat foods and eating more omega-3.

Slow-burn carbohydrates. We need the good carbohydrates, ones
that are slowly absorbed by the body. Limit the bad carbohydrates that
cause insulin and blood glucose spikes because they cause inflammation
and fat deposition. About one-half of our diet is derived from carbohydrates. The main purpose they serve is to provide fuel for the body and
brain, and they're fundamental to blood glucose sugar control.

For successful nutrition management, you should know the good
carbohydrates, which can be called *slow-burn carbs* because they don't
cause blood glucose, insulin spikes, or cortisol release – all of which can
lead to inflammation and life-threatening diseases.

It's also important to learn about the *glycemic index and glycemic load,*
which is a number given to foods based on how slowly or how quickly the
foods cause increases in blood glucose levels. The number is determined
by measuring the blood glucose after giving a person a specific food and
measuring the blood glucose level for a period of time afterward.

A high glycemic index means the food causes a high glucose level,
resulting in an insulin spike, and a low glycemic index means the food
causes no increase in blood glucose.

Low glycemic food is a source of energy; high glycemic food can
cause fat storage and synthesis of triglycerides, causing inflamed arteries.

Some high glycemic foods include baked goods, highly refined foods, white bread, mashed white potatoes, french fries, and white rice.

The dangerous insulin-surge effect of high glycemic foods can be countered by eating them along with foods containing protein, healthy fats, and fiber that can slow absorption, preventing the insulin spike.

The slow-burn complex carbohydrates are 20 or more sugar units chained together. Enzymes attack one end so they take a long time to break down, and therefore do not cause the insulin-surge response.

Fiber is a special carbohydrate. Although it may seem like eating cardboard, eating fiber is a powerful part of a nutritious diet. There are two types of fiber, soluble and insoluble, and they have multiple benefits. Fiber can make you feel full. It can maintain healthy blood sugar levels and prevent metabolic syndrome and prediabetes because it slows the absorption of sugar. And, the overall glycemic index is decreased, which prevents insulin surges.

Insoluble fiber is the woody portion of plant-based foods, such as broccoli and asparagus stems, and can regulate bowel function. These insoluble fibers can lower the risk of hemorrhoids, irritable bowel syndrome, and diverticulosis from less straining.

Soluble fiber is the gummy substance in oatmeal and red beans. It forms a gel with water, and beta-glucan in soluble fiber can decrease the blood level of low-density lipoprotein (LDL).

Fiber is important for people of all ages. Until age 50, men should get about 35 grams of fiber a day and women should get about 25; after age 50 the amount drops slightly, to about 30 grams for men and 20 for women. It's important to drink water when increasing fiber content because it can result in developing a *bezoar* ball in the stomach of a non-digestible substance, especially if a supplement such as psyllium is used too rapidly.

Eat fruits and vegetables with the peel. Add lentils and beans. Eat brown rice instead of white rice and eat high-fiber breakfast cereals for breakfast.

Want to lose weight? Ironically, diets are the biggest cause of weight gain in America. All types of diets can shed pounds of weight, but for how long? There is always the consequence of gaining 20 more pounds three to five years later. Ask anyone you know. Look it up.

The biggest cause of weight gain: lose 40 pounds with the latest diet and gain 50 pounds three years later.

We now know why this happens. Diets permanently slow the speed of metabolism.

Our brain has two nutrition systems. The hunger system determines how much to eat. The metabolism system determines the speed of metabolism, like a thermostat. The slower the metabolism, the less the amount of food is needed. During childhood and teenage years, these two systems are designed to be in balance, resulting in a healthy weight.

As people age, metabolism slows and muscle mass is lost, resulting in the need to eat less food. If people are able to eat healthy foods in the right quantity prepared in the right way during their lives, the hunger system slows at the same rate. These two systems stay in sync and result in a lifelong healthy weight.

However, beginning in the late teenage years, eating an unhealthy diet of added sugar, added salt, processed omega-6 fat, and too much saturated fats slows the metabolism system, but does not slow the hunger system.

The metabolism slows and less food is needed, but the hunger system doesn't change – sending messages to eat the same amount of food with the slower metabolism system. The leftover food piles up as fat around the belly and causes inflammation, diabetes, clogged arteries, and a shortened life.

Scientists have found out that diets do the same thing. Diets slow metabolism, but not the hunger system. As a result, people are just as hungry as before the diet, but the metabolism is slower, so the leftover calories per day gradually turn into 20 extra pounds over a few years.

There are potential solutions to fixing the problem of out-of-sync metabolism and hunger systems. All have unacceptable consequences except for one, which will be discussed after reviewing these not-so-good solutions.

Consider the issue of slow metabolism and how to speed it up. One way has been used for years and by millions of people – pills. Specifically, the amphetamines – they jazz up all of a person's body systems and result in loss of appetite and weight reduction.

The price? Much too high. First, it's an expensive pill that must be taken every day. Second, the adverse reactions are legendary and life-threating, including psychological dissociation; mental changes; blurred vision; dizziness; a false sense of well-being; a fast, irregular, pounding heartbeat; headache; restlessness; trouble sleeping; confusion; muscle cramps or spasms; seizures; vomiting; and loss of sexual ability, desire, drive, or performance. Third, as you would expect, as soon as the person stops taking the pills, their metabolism slows down again, and they rapidly return to their prior weight.

There will be newer speed-up-metabolism pills developed and maybe even based on natural substances with less adverse reactions; however, these alternatives are still going to be expensive, and a person will return to their baseline weight as soon as they stop taking the medication. These types of pills don't offer a useful, lifelong solution.

There are diets designed to speed up metabolism that may result in weight loss, but these designer diets are difficult to sustain and are often based on subtle calorie reduction that also may not be sustainable.

Let's look at the hunger system. How can we set it at a lower rate to match the slow metabolism rate? Hormonal pills. They are being developed to decrease the hunger system and likely with minimal adverse reactions, but once again, the daily cost and the need to continually take the pills to keep a balance does not provide a lifelong solution.

Let's hear about Olivia Fenston. Like too many people, she became obsessed with losing weight. She had gained 20 pounds during her college years and had not found a way to lose them.

She tried pills.

"Take one of these capsules and one of these tablets each morning," her doctor told her. The doctor also explained in detail the potential side effects, and warned her about one potentially life-threatening effect, but she wasn't listening. She had weight to lose and the pills were going to help.

She thought that everyone else was thin and beautiful, and she had to be the same way or she couldn't enjoy life. Yes, it was irrational and she knew it, but she didn't care. She had weight to lose.

"Look at the weight I'm losing," Olivia said to herself excitedly two weeks after starting on the pills. She had lost 15 pounds. "This is fantastic," she thought. "I'm going to be thin and beautiful."

Shortly afterward, however, she panicked when she felt a sharp pain in her right side just above the liver. She had heard about someone who had taken the same pills and had developed a severe side effect that required a lung transplant.

She rushed to see her doctor.

"Let's see what going on," the doctor said calmly. "It's probably a diaphragmatic muscle pull and not related to the pills."

"I don't care what it is," Olivia said frantically. "I'm not taking those pills. They'll kill me."

"That's a wise decision," the doctor said. "You look perfect just the way you are."

The doctor was right. We are all perfect just the way we are, but she didn't believe it and had to lose weight regardless of the dangers.

So Olivia started a vegetarian diet. However she failed to take the time to learn about the need for protein or to create a healthy diet plan. She believed that if she didn't consume meat or fish, she'd lose weight.

Two weeks later, she was cranky and irritable. She annoyed her friends by incessantly telling everyone about her diet, and she had gained two pounds. By three months, she was more frustrated than ever. Olivia had gained ten pounds! She also had a weakened immune system with inflamed skin lesions and prolonged recovery from colds.

How is this possible? It was obvious to everyone else. She had been eating pasta, cheese, and salads, and was stressed to the maximum. These foods contained added sugar, added salt, and too many processed omega-6 fats. These foods turn into storage fat, increasing weight. The stress triggered cortisol, which is a glucocorticoid steroid released by the adrenal glands, causing excessive blood sugar that is converted to abdominal fat.

Olivia was desperate. She hadn't lost weight from her previous gain of two pounds, and now she had gained another ten pounds.

She then heard about a miracle weight-loss guava juice that was made with a leafy vegetable grown in Southeast Asia. It was from an exotic location, and it was natural, so it had to work, she thought.

"Stop! Don't take that drink," Olivia's doctor said.

"Why not?"

"It can cause constrictive bronchiolitis."

"What? What'd you say?" Olivia asked. "I can't even pronounce it."

"That drink can cause some rare lung disease by scarring the small airways and can even cause death in really bad situations," her doctor answered. "It was banned in Southeast Asia."

"That's impossible. How can vegetable leaves cause a problem with the lungs?"

"It contains a toxin that attacks the airways."

"I'm glad you told me. Forget it. I'm not touching that drink."

So, Olivia signed up for a weight-loss spa advertised on television. The instructors taught her about metabolism and healthy nutrition, which was good, but she didn't really absorb any of the information. The program also included an exercise program, but to Olivia, it was too much work.

She attended a mind-body institute weight-loss program, but it didn't work for her because she kept falling asleep.

Meanwhile, Olivia was so stressed about trying to lose weight that she gained another ten pounds.

Several years later, Olivia had failed to find the right program and reached the obesity range. She developed diabetes and hypertension, and continued to feel that everyone was so thin and beautiful and that she wasn't. She developed severe depression and lost her job.

———

Unfortunately, similar sad stories are repeated too often among people all over the world. People feel they must lose weight, whether it's 20 pounds or 100 pounds, and obsession takes over their lives. They search for pills, for diets, for anything that will easily make the weight go away, failing to realize that the solution lies within themselves. To lose weight and keep it off, they need to develop a successful *lifelong* program.

Nutrition is a complex science about how the interaction of different foods affects our health. The process of developing a program begins with learning everything possible about nutrition.

———

Wendy Martin gained 20 pounds during her college years, but really didn't pay attention to the increase in weight and had no ambition about trying to look thin or beautiful like the women in magazines and on television.

She felt good about herself, but eventually realized her flabby belly wasn't attractive and decided to eliminate it. She had only gained 20 pounds, but knew that it may take two or three years to lose it, and that it wouldn't be an easy, one-step fix.

Wendy began with the first step. She learned about nutrition. She bought a CD and listened to it during her 30-minute drive to work. She visited academic websites and learned about carbohydrate metabolism and abdominal fat. She learned about fat and protein metabolism, and vitamins and minerals. She even learned about water and hydration.

Wendy had heard about the dangers of diet pills, and after studying the different types, concluded that some of them were effective in the short term, but the potential side effects were not worth the risk.

"How should I approach the situation?" Wendy asked a sports nutritionist.

"First, continue your positive approach and keep learning," the nutritionist said. "You have developed a good beginning by approaching nutrition with an attitude that will lead to success.

"Second step, let's take a nutrition inventory."

Wendy recorded her height and weight. From these two values, she calculated her body mass index, or BMI, which was 28.5 – not too high but above the normal level of 25. She measured her waist circumference, and calculated her body fat percentage, which was 22 percent – again, not too high, but also above the healthy level.

Wendy and her nutritionist calculated how many calories and the volume of water she needed on a daily basis. To complete the inventory, her blood pressure, her fasting blood sugar, and her kidney function were measured as baselines to ensure that she had not developed early signs of excessive weight-related medical conditions such as diabetes or hypertension.

"This is great," Wendy said. "I really know where I stand, and I now have a basis to go forward."

"That's the second step," the nutritionist said. "Now, let's look at the third step – the management options."

"I've read about diet pills," Wendy said. "There seem to be different types. Some suppress appetite. Some ramp up the body to burn extra calories. Some claim to manipulate hormones. But none are for me. They have too many potentially dangerous side effects, and they're not permanent solutions."

"Let's talk about diets," the nutritionist said. "There are millions of them."

"I found out they're like pills," Wendy said. "Follow a list of specific foods. If you stop, the weight returns just like the pills."

"But, some diets have good components," the nutritionist said, "such as foods that have low saturated fat, low sugar, low sodium, or high fiber. Diets can help some people."

"For me, they're too complicated," Wendy said, "they're not a lifetime solution because foods change over time and our metabolism efficiency changes over time."

"You've done your homework, the nutritionist replied. "Specific diets for diseases can be useful short term, but we're talking about a lifelong program."

"So," Wendy said, "now that we've discussed pills and diets, what's left?"

"You develop a nutrition plan that's best for you," the nutritionist said. "It's the *what, when, how,* and *where* answers that work."

Wendy learned the answers to these questions that were right for her. She used her personal nutrition monitors and soon returned to her healthy weight, which boosted her energy and enthusiasm for life.

She understood her nutrition. She ate foods prepared in a healthy way in the right amounts at the right times.

————

We have two stories, each of which tells us about 20 extra pounds. Does either one apply to you?

Olivia is a wonderful person but did everything wrong. She became obsessed with losing weight. She failed to learn about nutrition. She failed to learn about her body's nutritional status. She hoped that pills and diets would lead to a solution, but didn't know that she was so stressed out from wanting to lose weight that, paradoxically, these methods didn't work because the stress released more cortisol, creating increased fat storage. Importantly, she wasn't being herself. She wanted to be someone else – a thin person she saw in magazines and on TV.

Wendy did it correctly. She approached her weight loss in a positive manner. She learned about nutrition. She asked questions and understood the answers. She took a nutritional inventory. Wendy took charge of her nutrition and found a solution.

––––

Here's another story about making wrong healthy food choices. Brad complained to a nutritionist that he continued to gain weight even though he'd been eating nothing. The nutritionist didn't believe it until Brad explained the details. He wasn't eating anything solid, but he was drinking his food and in a surprisingly large amount – five huge 30- to 40-ounce containers of sodas and fruit "smoothies" every day.

A 32-ounce sugar cola may contain 310 calories, but one supersized, 40-ounce ice-cream fruit smoothie can have an astounding 1,500 calories! You do the math. Brad was drinking five sodas and smoothies – 4,000 to 6,000 calories a day. It won't take long to pack on the pounds.

Furthermore, the amount of sugar, saturated fats, and processed omega-6 can be astronomical in sodas and ice cream smoothies, which can rapidly cause inflamed, clogged arteries and cardiovascular disease.

––––

How can you take charge of your nutrition?

Dave and Kelly were talking about diets and food during their lunch break. "I need your advice," Dave said. "I've got to lose this extra 20 pounds around my belly. What should I do?"

"Whoa, you're asking me?" Kelly asked jokingly.

"Yup. You look trim and healthy, so I'm sure you can help me. I've tried pills and diets. The pills are too dangerous. The diets are too confusing and have too many rules, and I was annoying everyone and myself by always talking about being on a diet. Besides, I couldn't follow any of them long enough to help. What'd you do?"

"It's hard work," Kelly said, "but not impossible. I put in the work and the food works for me. I learned everything I could about nutrition. This is what I found: eat the right food in the right amount at the right time, and it'll take care of you forever!"

"That sounds nice. But what do you mean?"

"Eat the right foods – slow-burn carbohydrates like vegetables, whole grains, and fiber, fats like omega-3 foods, and lean protein," Kelly said. "Eat the right amount, too – learn the food thresholds. All foods are good. It's going over the threshold amount that's bad – eat over the threshold and some foods will cause inflamed arteries and fat bellies."

"What's a food threshold?" Dave asked.

"At a certain low level no food is dangerous, even the toxic puffer fish, but above that level, that puffer fish can kill you," Kelly said dramatically. "Many types of common carbohydrates and foods containing saturated fats have low threshold levels, especially processed foods and sugary drinks. Try eating one french fry or one potato chip, or one sip of a smoothie?" Kelly shook her head. "It's so easy to go over the risk threshold with these foods that I completely avoid them most days, and that strategy works for me. Fortunately, there are many healthy foods – like spinach, vegetables, and omega-3 foods – that have such high thresholds you can eat much more of them and be safe."

"So, you're saying to keep healthy," Dave said, "I should eat the right foods in the right amounts, and they will protect my blood vessels and my heart, and also provide the high energy I need to have an exciting, productive day."

"You got it! That's it," Kelly said as they returned to work.

Listen to your "belly brain." It's trying to tell you something. Everyone has a belly brain. It's very much like a second brain. It's called the *enteric nervous system* – the separate but interconnected nervous system that works along your entire intestinal tract, your mouth, and to a lesser extent, your gallbladder and pancreas. There are as many neurons in your enteric nervous system as in your spinal cord, which gives the system the ability to convey a massive amount of information.

Science has known about the enteric nervous system for more than a hundred years, but most of us still perceive the brain in our heads as being in control of our bodies. In fact, at the subconscious level, more information passes from your belly brain to your head brain than vice versa. If you're surprised by that, consider such established adages in Western culture as having a "gut feeling" about something or someone. In many Eastern cultures also, people will tap their stomachs when they're asked where they think.

Let's listen to our belly brain for a minute.

Think in your mind about eating a greasy food dripping with fat. How does your stomach react? Now think about a banana. How does your stomach react?

That's the belly brain talking to you. It may not speak English or in full sentences, but it's definitely giving you an opinion. You may not want to believe it, but that's a distressed "no" for the greasy food and a calming "yes" for the banana.

There are some people whose mouth may be watering at the thought of a greasy stack of french fries and fat dripping from a steak at the conscious level, but at the belly brain and the subconscious are squirming with unhealthy distress.

Why does the belly brain have to be so powerful? The gut has to assess everything we take into our bodies and figure out what to do with it. What part of what we've eaten is vitamins? What part is made up of other nutrients? What part is fuel? How much insulin does the pancreas need to make? How much bile is needed from the gallbladder? Should our body use what's coming in immediately or save it for a time when it would be better to digest? Is something we've taken in a threat or a toxin?

These seem like straightforward issues to address, but they're complex. Nutritionists acknowledge that they don't know how everything works together, but a few dynamics between what we take in and how our bodies use it have become clear.

One important dynamic is the interplay between stress and digestion. Insulin, the hormone made by the pancreas, works to push sugar into cells from the bloodstream.

When we're relaxed and our calming parasympathetic nervous system pathways dominate, we make the right amount of insulin to digest what we eat. But when we're stressed, our hyped-up sympathetic nervous system takes over, and cortisol is the hormone activated. We not only signal our digestion to move more slowly or come to a halt, we make more insulin and the cortisol level goes up. When the body feels high stress constantly, these two hormones work together to store fat and add weight. And that high cortisol causes inflammation.

High cortisol levels influence the cephalic, or head phase, of digestion, which accounts for about 40 to 60 percent of total digestion. The cephalic phase includes sensory details gleaned from taste, aroma, visual appreciation of food, and our pleasure from it. When we're looking forward to a meal and smelling it as it cooks, our mouths water in anticipation, readying our bodies to take in all those nutrients.

For some people, anticipation of a meal is such a powerful thing that they start producing insulin just thinking about it, which is called the cephalic phase insulin response.

But when we're stressed and the excitable sympathetic nervous system dominates, cortisol desensitizes our bodies to pleasure, whether it's touch or taste. As we decrease our ability to taste or anticipate and experience pleasure from a meal, we inhibit our ability to get the nutrients we need from our food. Eventually, we're going to need to eat more, which means our bodies need to produce more insulin.

All those extra calories consumed cause insulin surges that not only result in weight gain but can also lead to cellular inflammation.

Our emotions and certain psychological archetypes also influence how we approach eating and our cephalic phase. Sometimes we act like children who eat for comfort. Sometimes we see ourselves as victims and think that we might as well overeat because no one will love us whether we're thin or heavy. Sometimes we might play the rebel and say, "I'll eat what I want, and who are you to tell me differently?" Sometimes we are wolves who devour our food. And sometimes we're cold scientists who regard food as fuel and nothing else.

Unfortunately, though, the fat that is deposited from eating under stress usually goes right to the middle. We can feel increased bloating, indigestion, and damaging gastrointestinal reflux.

But before you think you're in thrall to your belly brain, remember that your head brain can influence the system, too. If stress deprives you of nutrients and causes weight gain, and all the problems that go with that, you can take concrete steps to give better signals to your belly brain.

Ask yourself if you're about to eat while stressed. If the answer is yes, try to figure out why. Start with: *Who's eating? The rebel? The child?* Pretend instead that you're a healthy, strong person who eats in a dignified, self-respecting manner.

In addition to this sort of visualization, try to take three to five belly breaths to fool your belly brain into thinking you're calm. A belly breath moves your lower abdomen outward with each deep breath. Or play some music. Focus one of your senses on something calming, like candles, palm trees, or a soft, sandy beach.

You should try an ancient yogic technique, which is to eat only until you've reached "thermic" efficiency. This means to eat until your body has taken in enough fuel to satisfy your energy needs, which is a feeling you can train your mind to sense, just before you start to feel full.

Eat to your high-energy level, not to your overly full level.

Most important of all, slow down while you eat. Your body considers food that's consumed too fast a stressor all by itself. You might have heard of the French paradox: even though the French diet consists of more fat per person per year than the diet of Americans and other cultures, the French on average show lower rates of diabetes, obesity, and cardiovascular disease.

Researchers found that red wine was the advantage. It's the color red. There is also a benefit from colorful foods such as grapes, cranberries, blueberries, purple eggplant and orange peppers. But nutritionists believe that French people generally take pleasure in their food. They tend to eat longer and more relaxed meals at midday, which is a time when the body is programmed to digest and extract all the nutrients from food most efficiently. In fact, you can optimize weight loss and calorie-burning by taking advantage of this natural body rhythm and eating the majority of your calories in the first half of the day.

A breakfast is especially useful because the belly brain reacts by digesting the food efficiently, smoothing out the insulin surges and not storing fat. If you're eating at ten at night, you're not burning calories efficiently, which can result in fat deposition, and you're not giving your digestive system the nightly time of repair and rejuvenation.

Cook foods in the right way. Foods cooked at extremely high temperatures that are fried, barbecued, or broiled can result in foods containing glycation end-products. This glycation process occurs when glucose and proteins in foods are fused together and produce aberrant end products. These substances are not recognized naturally by our digestive system and can't be metabolized efficiently. The higher the saturated fat content in these foods, the higher the glycation rate is going to be from high-temperature cooking.

Glycation end-products are also found in some packaged foods such as preheated products or frozen precooked meals.

These poorly metabolized substances, sometimes termed *glycotoxins,* can cause cellular inflammation throughout the body organs and especially the internal walls of the blood vessels, which can result in cardiovascular disease.

Diabetics are especially vulnerable to these effects. Diabetics who have high levels of glycation end-products may develop heart, kidney, or eye complications, while those who maintain low levels often do not. It is interesting to note, though, that a small percentage of diabetics with high levels of glycation end-products do not develop complications, which may mean these individuals have a genetically-enabled enzyme to neutralize these toxic substances.

Steaming and slow, low-heat cooking minimize glycation substances.

Artificial sweeteners do not qualify as high-quality foods. For one thing, they have no nutritional value. They provide a sweet taste and nothing else, and no studies have shown that they help people lose weight. Worse, people may consume excessive amounts of foods that contain these artificial sweeteners, such as diet sodas, resulting in gum disease and tooth decay from the acidic carbonation.

The sweet taste in some artificial sweeteners activates the sweet taste buds in the tongue that could result in an insulin surge. That surge may cause hypoglycemia because there is no new source of glucose, so this extra insulin triggers cortisol release, inflammation, and fat storage.

Nina learned about this. She had two big diet sodas for breakfast every day and wondered why she was dizzy, irritable, and cranky an hour or so later. Her blood sugar had plummeted to 55, when it should be around 80.

Lifelong healthy eating. Eat healthy foods in the right quantity, at the right time, and prepared in the right way. Use mindful eating. Chew all the bites and eat slowly. Eat without stress or tension. Stop eating when you have the feeling from signals that you've eaten enough.

After a reasonable amount of food, stop eating and take a 20-minute break, if you are still hungry, eat some more, but almost all of the time you will have the feeling of fullness and won't need to eat any more. This is because of the leptin/ghrelin system. As discussed earlier, leptin is the hormone produced by fat cells when there has been sufficient amount of food eaten and ghrelin is produced by the intestinal cells when additional food is needed. This system is slow – it takes about 20 minutes for the cells to send the leptin signal to the brain to stop eating.

Regarding ghrelin, this signal of a growling stomach and the feeling of being hungry can be strong, but know that this is a signal to eat food, not a signal to eat a large amount of food. This is why during Thanksgiving dinner, you stop eating when you have the feeling of being full – which is 20 minutes too late. Being overly full is going to send you to the couch with a bloated, stuffed stomach and feeling terrible. It's a slow system.

Healthy nutrition is a lifestyle, not a diet: no added sugar, no added salt, and no processed omega-6 fats. Added sugar, added salt, and processed omega-6 fats cause inflammation, which in turn causes inflammatory-based diseases, including heart disease, strokes, hypertension, diabetes, and cancer.

How do you live a no-added sugar, no added salt, and no processed omega-6 lifestyle? Look at the ingredient list on labels. If sugar and sodium salt are listed, find another food. To stay clear of processed omega-6 fats, avoid ultra-processed foods and farm-raised fish, poultry, and beef.

There's no need to tell anyone you are doing this. It's annoying for other people, and Americans have been so conditioned to the taste of sugar and salt in the diet that people won't want to hear negative comments about these two additives.

There are three issues that you will encounter when you stop eating foods with added sugar, added salt, and processed omega-6 fats.

First, sugar is addicting, so you will likely dream about hot-fudge sundaes and other desserts or may have other minor withdrawal symptoms. This is not a big issue and quickly fades over a few days.

Second, you need to maintain this lifestyle. To do this, you need to recruit your subconscious mind. Some foods may be bland and tasteless at first because you're not use to them. Try a new non-harmful food at least three times.

You need to condition the subconscious mind with positive reinforcement to make the right food choices. You do this by thinking about the lifelong positive emotional feeling of good health from eating foods that are not going to harm you and contrast this to the two minutes of pleasure you'll get from a yummy dessert – which will be followed by the crash from eating sugar foods.

It's a long-term health benefit versus a short-term pleasure issue. It's boring versus exciting. Will power is not enough. You need to recruit your subconscious mind.

Use your subconscious mind and prefrontal cortex as a positive loop for eating these healthy foods. If you're hungry, and you eat a healthy snack like an apple, the feeling of no longer being hungry will send a dopamine surge to the accumbens pleasure center, which in turn will send a signal to the prefrontal lobe registering this as a positive event. If this is repeated three or more times, you will most likely continue to eat this food, and you may even develop a craving for this healthy food.

For example, we have eaten oatmeal with added sugar and added salt since childhood. And our parents and grandparents have eaten oatmeal with these additives. So, we are well conditioned to recognize this taste associated with oatmeal, but these two inflammatory-causative additives are harmful.

Try this: purchase organic oats from the farmland with no other ingredients. Add water and warm. Your first taste does not recognize it as oatmeal. It is bland with a pasty consistency. But if you're hungry and add blueberries, your subconscious accumbens registers pleasure and sends a positive message to the prefrontal cortex. Try it a second and third time – your conscious mind begins to enjoy the subtle tastes and texture because the prefrontal lobe has made a positive association. Who knows, you may even develop a craving for this no-sugar, no-salt oatmeal.

The third issue with this no added sugar, no added salt, and no processed omega-6 lifestyle is a social one. It's not easy to find these foods. Currently, there is no section in the supermarket designated for no added sugar and no added salt, making it difficult to find foods such as breads, bagels, spaghetti sauce, canned beans, canned fruit, and vegan food. You have to read the labels and once you find the right foods, stick with them.

The other social issue is what to do when faced with having a piece of birthday cake at the office or dessert for a celebration. You can say you ate too much or you'll have it later, but a healthy option is to go ahead and enjoy the celebration without making people uncomfortable and feeling guilty because a small amount of added sugar on occasion is not harmful.

This is a lifestyle, not a diet, so you're not breaking rules. No need to be stressed, feel guilty, or beat yourself up. It's a celebration, enjoy the cake or dessert and enjoy the company. The digestion system is not under stress and the positive effect of the event will outweigh the negative effect of a small amount of extra sugar.

These are the three issues, what about the benefits?

The first thing that happens is that you feel good about yourself because you're not eating foods that are going to harm you. It feels wonderful to have no anxiety or guilt associated with eating. Your food choices are not going to harm you and may even help you.

Second, you may lose your belly fat, resulting in a flat stomach, which indicates a decrease in the inflammatory-based diseases.

Third, you are decreasing the lifelong risk of heart disease, strokes, hypertension, diabetes, and cancer.

The no added sugar, no added salt, and no processed omega-6 lifestyle may be difficult at first, but over time it becomes a habit, and these healthy foods will eventually become more widely available and easier to find in the grocery store.

Lifelong healthy nutrition means eating the right food, prepared in a healthy manner, in the right amount, and at the right time.

CHAPTER 9
SLEEP: YOU NEED
EIGHT HOURS

Sleep eight hours every day. You need eight, not six and not ten. There are two reasons for eight hours: to restore your brain adenosine and to get the required amount of REM (rapid-eye movement) sleep.

Science has taught us the energy chemical in the brain called *adenosine* is gradually depleted during the day's activities. Eight hours of sleep is needed to restore the balance of adenosine. Five is not enough and ten is too much. Choose a time to go to bed, add eight hours, and get up, not before and not after.

You can take a daytime nap but only for 15 minutes or less – anything longer will reset your natural sleep pattern and you won't sleep at night.

Finally, do not fall asleep watching television.

The function of sleep remained a mystery for centuries, but now, we have begun to find answers to explain our unrivaled need for sleep. Simply stated, it's not to rest the body, it's for the brain. Sleep recharges the brain, and it takes eight hours to do this.

———

Mark put his laptop down on his cubicle desk with a thump and an angry sigh.

"Was it rough in there?" his friend Jeff asked from a nearby desk. Jeff knew Mark had just given a presentation to their boss.

"Brutal," Mark said. "They asked me question after question, way too quickly, and it was clear they think I hadn't thought the whole thing through, which is crazy. I worked hard staying up late for the past three nights getting ready for this."

"And thanks for helping me after I ran in here late," he added.

"No problem," Jeff said. "What happened, by the way? You oversleep?"

"I fell asleep on the train and missed the stop. Then I had to wait for another train going in the other direction."

"That's happened to everyone, I'm sure," Jeff said, although it had never happened to him.

Mark shuffled some papers, knocking a few off his desk. "And it'll probably happen again tomorrow, too, because I've got to figure out how to make this project work. I'll be up all night again," he said, angrily.

"Try some sleep, it'll give you energy to finish the project," Jeff said without trying to lecture his friend.

"Who has time?"

"Who doesn't is the better question. Sleep is important. Healthy sleep allows you to come up with good ideas, boosts your mood, and gives you the energy to tackle all the things they" – Jeff pointed toward the conference room – "toss at you."

Mark sat down heavily. "I've never needed a lot of sleep. I can fall asleep in two minutes anytime I want and anyplace."

"That's a bad sign. It's not a good thing," Jeff said. "You just flunked the five-minute sleep test – you're chronically sleep deprived."

"What's the five-minute sleep test?" Mark asked.

"Sit quietly for five minutes without distractions. If you fall asleep before five minutes is up, you flunk and you have sleep deprivation."

"That doesn't sound good."

"Worse yet, if this happens to you at several times during the month, you now have chronic sleep deprivation," Jeff explained with concern.

"What happens then?" Mark asked.

"You know what happens," Jeff replied. "At first you continually feel angry and upset about every little thing. Then you start to blame others, criticize, and make excuses. Then comes depression. Finally over time, inflammation develops from the stress toxins causing heart disease, hypertension, strokes, cancer, and death." Jeff added dramatically.

"Not a pretty picture," commented Mark.

———

The way Mark thinks about sleep is all too common. There is so much competing for our attention and time that sleep can seem like a waste of time.

People brag about only needing five hours of sleep. They have convinced themselves of this, but they don't realize they're only functioning at 60 percent of their potential productivity and thinking ability. Don't boast about not needing eight hours of sleep – everyone needs it.

Performance tests have determined that cognitive abilities like memory and concentration decrease markedly when people get less than seven hours of sleep a night. During sleep, the brain forms and reinforces memories of tasks learned. Without adequate sleep, it takes longer to learn and remember.

The ability to concentrate, focus, and stay on task suffers with too little sleep, especially too little REM sleep. Researchers call this "ability vigilance" and test it by asking a person to press a button when a light dot randomly appears on a screen. The test focuses on measuring how many times the person realizes the dot is there and presses the button, assessing how often the person's attention stays on the screen or strays from it.

A person who slept less than seven hours performs much worse on the vigilance test than someone who slept for eight hours. A person who sleeps six hours or less a day misses a much greater number of dots, and if that sleep pattern is maintained for two weeks, the scores will continue to decline.

And worse, the person loses creativity and is not aware of it. We all know that after a night of little, no, or very poor sleep, we can get grumpy. But, the sleep deprivation of having six hours of sleep or less per day gives a person a new sense of "normal." In this state, a person might not make the best choices, from what foods to eat for lunch, to arguing with a spouse over a minor annoyance, to taking a curve at 50 miles per hour instead of the recommended 25.

If this description sounds like someone who has been drinking too much alcohol, you're right. Researchers have compared sleep deprivation to alcohol intoxication levels and found a direct correlation – the more sleep deprived a person is, the stronger that person compares to someone with an increased blood alcohol level.

Most of our jobs don't require that we concentrate all the time, so they don't provide feedback about whether we've entered a period of consistent sleep deprivation. We can force ourselves to perform well when called on, but often we're performing on autopilot, and when sleep deprived, this is about 60 percent of our full capability, and this level of autopilot can have bad consequences.

The Exxon Valdez oil spill disaster has been attributed, not to rare, bizarre circumstances, but to fatigue of the captain, who had been working at least 18 hours before the ship ran aground.

You don't have to be driving a large oil tanker to be affected. The National Transportation Safety Board attributes about 30 percent of fatal accidents on the country's freeways to driver fatigue.

Sleeping less than eight hours a day can also contribute to long-term health consequences. Lack of sleep and sleep deprivation is a stressor to the body's organ systems, including the heart and metabolism. Your body's ability to regulate blood glucose levels is sharply decreased by sleep deprivation.

The less sleep you have, the higher your blood glucose, which could result in insulin resistance, increased fat deposition, and diabetes. Increased fat deposition from sleep deprivation is due to increased ghrelin, the appetite hormone, and decreased leptin, the appetite-suppressor hormone.

That's what happens when we don't get eight hours of sleep.

So why do we need eight hours? The energy chemical adenosine needs to be recharged and the required REM sleep needs to occur during the seventh and eighth hour of sleep time.

In the past sleep has been considered necessary to rest the body. There is no information to suggest that the body needs sleep. Now the sleep requirement is placed squarely in the brain. It's the brain that needs sleep.

A group of nerves or neurons located in the frontal lobe of the brain use the substance adenosine as their energy source, and these neurons are highly active during the day. As the neurons fire to send signals among themselves, they leave adenosine behind. This chemical builds up in the space between the neurons and some of it binds to a receptor on the surface of the neurons. The more adenosine that binds to these receptors, the less the neurons can fire. Eventually, the surface of the neurons becomes covered with adenosine, stopping the functioning of the neurons and your clear thinking.

This is where the eight hours comes in. It takes eight hours to clear the adenosine and restore balance.

There's a reason that caffeine keeps people awake. Caffeine is an anti-adenosine chemical. Caffeine stops the adenosine from binding to the neuron surface. But this is only temporary; no matter how much coffee or other caffeine energy drinks you consume, eventually you must sleep to restore the adenosine balance and recharge the brain. We've all experienced the feeling of being both wide awake and exhausted at the same time. That's the brain telling you it needs to restore balance.

Again, the first reason you need eight hours of sleep is to restore the balance of adenosine and the second reason has to do with REM sleep, which is rapid eye movement sleep related to dreaming. Research findings have shown that at least 90 minutes of REM sleep is required for optimal health and productivity. This REM dreaming period is a time when the brain organizes the day's events making neuro-connections with past events. If you wake up during this time, you may discover a solution to a lingering problem.

The key finding for the eight-hour sleep requirement is that almost all of the REM sleep occurs during the last two to three hours of sleep before awakening in the morning. This is why someone can see your eyes moving quickly before you get up. You need these last two hours of sleep to attain that REM requirement – one more meaningful reason you need eight hours of sleep and not five or six hours.

These last two-hours of the eight-hour sleep provides the positive qualities of being human. This REM sleep enables the qualities of kindness, gratitude, thinking about others, creativity, and grace. Without these last two hours, negative traits dominate that include irritability, being temperamental, anger, depression, self-centered, and minimal positive engagement in other people's lives. These last two hours are needed for the joy of life.

So what are some tried-and-true steps to getting the sleep you need?

Since caffeine stimulates the brain and keeps it going when the brain wants to come back to balance, limit your caffeine intake late in the day. Get plenty of exercise. Eat well. Avoid alcohol before bedtime. Reduce noise, distractions, and temperature fluctuations as best as you can. Try not to bring whatever's worrying you to bed. Use your mind to clear recurring negative thoughts.

One of the biggest mistakes people make is falling asleep for 30 minutes to an hour while watching TV at eight or nine o'clock at night. A midday 15-minute nap can be beneficial, but the evening TV nap is deadly. You'll find yourself tossing and turning all night.

But you can change the habit. First, a little background: bright lights help us set our circadian clock, our bodies' daily rhythms. Therefore it's helpful to limit exposure to bright lights – especially computer and mobile device screens – before going to bed. It's also helpful to go to bed at the same time every night, add eight hours, and then get out of bed. Not less and not more than eight hours. Doing this keeps your circadian clock in rhythm with the body's natural balance.

Keep in mind that assigning labels like "morning person" or "night owl" can be hazardous. They can set you up for trouble. For example, "I'm not a morning person" or "Don't talk to me in the morning" are myth statements. They set up a neurolinguistic conditioning cycle that, with belief and practice, becomes true. Consider that there is no such thing as a morning person or a night owl.

There are several ways to help you fall asleep once in bed. Read something that's not demanding for a few minutes. Or try the countdown method: begin at 100 and slowly count backward to 90 and repeat as needed. Often you'll fall asleep before reaching 90 the first time and almost always after several times.

Another option is to use self-hypnotic muscle relaxation: begin with your toes, relaxing each one of them; then proceed to your feet, ankles, calves, and knees; moving through the abdomen, chest, arms, neck, and finally the head, deeply relaxing each area of your body. Use your breathing to make this relaxation technique more effective – silently breathe in and out equally without making a sound and remembering to move your lower abdomen up with each in-breath. Use yoga breathing, equal breath in to equal breath out.

If these sleep-inducing methods don't work and you're still experiencing disrupted or fragmented sleep, then there's a possibility that a health condition, such as sleep apnea, restless leg movements, hormonal fluctuations, or pain, could be responsible for your trouble. Some sleeping problems do require a visit to the doctor. Talk to your doctor about your sleep issues, especially if you're experiencing insomnia and cannot get to sleep at all.

But above all, give yourself the time in bed. Some people sleep right through the night. Others sleep in a couple of chunks, waking up for a while before falling asleep again. Others nap for 15 minutes in the midafternoon. All of these are normal patterns. What matters is that you find what works best for you so that you feel "charged up" for the next day.

It's important to use the bed for sleeping only. This means no watching TV in bed and especially no watching videos on a mobile device, because the brain gets use to these activities, and they're not counted toward the eight hours of sleep. In addition, blue light from the screens strikes the retina eye receptors, which causes a decrease in melatonin release from the brain, further delaying sleep.

You need eight hours of naturally occurring sleep to restore the high-energy brain-cell balance necessary for a successful day. Stimulants and artificial means of interfering with this natural brain restoration will only serve to change an exciting, high-energy day to a weak, low-energy one.

———

After completing his annual physical examination, Dave asked his doctor a question about sleep.

"I can't sleep. Could you give me some sleeping pills or let me take melatonin?" Dave pleaded.

"Tell me about your sleep pattern."

"What do you mean?"

"What time do you go to sleep at night? When do you wake up? Do you fall asleep during the day or evening?" Dr. Anderson asked.

"I never thought about it. Every day is different."

"This may be the problem."

"Why? What difference does it make?" Dave asked.

"The brain needs a natural sleep pattern," Dr. Anderson explained. "It requires the same pattern every day to restore the energy chemical balance and to get the required amount of REM sleep."

"What's REM sleep?" Dave asked. "And how much of it do we need?"

"It's rapid-eye movement sleep, and we need at least 90 minutes of REM sleep," the doctor explained. "Importantly, the REM sleep occurs during the last two hours of the eight-hour sleep requirement."

"I've never heard of that," Dave replied. "So that's why I have to have eight hours of sleep?"

"Yes, that's one reason," answered the doctor, "And, eight hours of sleep is needed to balance the adenosine energy chemical."

"That's complicated, but sounds like two good reasons to get eight hours of sleep," Dave said, finally understanding.

"Now, tell me about your sleep pattern," the doctor said.

"I can tell you about yesterday. It was a typical Wednesday: I came home from work, had a great dinner with Kate, and we watched a TV show we both liked. We had some peanuts and a beer during the show. We didn't bother to change the channel afterward and fell asleep about nine and woke up an hour later."

"Anything else?"

"I was still hungry so I snacked on something from the refrigerator, and we went to bed after midnight. My eyes were wide open and I couldn't sleep. That's why I need your help."

"When did you need to get up for work?"

"I had an early-morning meeting, so the alarm went off a few minutes before six."

"Sounds like five or six hours of sleep," Dr. Anderson said. "You need eight, and that late one hour of snoozing in front of the TV was more disruptive than beneficial. It was way too close to bedtime. The snack you had at midnight also kept you awake."

"I didn't realize these bad habits were affecting my sleep," Dave said.

"A lot of people make these same mistakes," the doctor said. "You don't need sleeping pills. You need to establish a good, consistent sleep pattern."

"Sounds boring," Dave said. But feeling curious and desperate, he asked, "How do I do it?"

"Go to bed at the same time every night, add eight hours, and get up."

"That's sounds like a good start," Dave said. "I won't fall asleep before going to bed."

"Good. Is there anything else you can think of doing or not doing that might help with your sleep pattern?" the doctor asked.

"How about not eating or drinking anything three hours before I go to sleep?" Dave asked.

"That's the answer," Dr. Anderson said. "It'll take you awhile, but if you stick with it most nights, it'll pay huge rewards."

Although it did take some time, Dave and Kate both developed healthy sleep patterns and noticed great improvement in their energy levels. They quickly forgot about their TV snoozes and midnight snacks. The trick was taping their favorite TV shows so they could watch them whenever they wanted.

Obtain your eight hours of sleep every night for a long, healthy, and vigorous life.

CHAPTER 10
EXERCISE: YOU MIGHT
MEET YOUR SPOUSE

There are more than 100 positive reasons for one hour of daily exercise. My top three include exercise gives you energy, decreases stress, and produces feel-good neurotransmitters and hormones. And, randomly, you might meet your spouse.

One hour of continuous exercise every day will give you the energy needed to get through the day. This is counterintuitive, but one of the best reasons to exercise. This amount of exercise produces the feel-good neurotransmitters and hormones such as endorphins, dopamine, and serotonin.

Exercising together in a group class such as spinning, body pump, or dance produces oxytocin, the bonding hormone. Numerous studies have proven that exercise reduces stress, increases conditioning, and improves concentration. Exercise makes you feel better.

Here's a myth: exercise makes you tired. In fact, it's the opposite. Exercise gives you energy. The more exercise you do up to one hour, the more energy you'll have.

Exercise of just about any type can be beneficial. Try all of them and mix them up. You can exercise in the morning, after work, or whenever you please. You can exercise at a workout facility, a gym, a community center, or at home. You can exercise alone or with a group.

It's important to remember that regardless of the exercise, it needs to be performed regularly, and correct form is fundamental. Let's explore how exercise can provide you with energy.

Exercise increases energy across almost all population groups, and improves mood even in the absence of fitness improvements. This means that for the most sedentary people, a short spurt of 20 minutes of easy exercise, such as a brisk walk, swimming, or yoga, can be effective.

What about fatigue? Did you know that one-quarter of the population reports persistent fatigue? For sedentary people with a low fitness level, the good news is that all it takes is some low-intensity exercise for improvement of fatigue symptoms – like taking a 20-minute walk every day. It's an excellent way to decrease fatigue for sedentary people, helping them to feel better and become more active. The reason is this: the body and mind respond favorably to simple movement.

So, how does exercise improve energy? The body responds immediately when a person starts exercising. The heart and lungs begin to work, bringing more oxygen and nutrients to cells and carrying away toxins. The powerhouse mitochondria, which are the energy-producing centers of the cells, go into accelerated action. The body's core temperature warms up, increasing chemical reactions. More blood flow goes to the working muscles, improving the transfer of oxygen and nutrients.

Mental clarity improves as the brain responds by increasing the energy and feel-good neurotransmitters norepinephrine, dopamine, and serotonin. Exercise is a natural way to generate these neurotransmitters, which are the same chemicals used as many antidepressant drugs. Strenuous long-duration exercise such as running, swimming, biking, and even yoga produce endorphins, which reduce our perception of pain, decrease stress, and produce a feeling of well-being.

The one-time occurrence of exercise provides increased energy as an acute response, while daily exercise provides the benefits of persistent energy and improved fitness as a chronic response.

Increasing your fitness level through exercise means the body becomes more efficient, basal metabolism is increased, muscles become stronger, and exercise becomes easier. The most exciting improvement that accompanies increased fitness is having more energy, being creative, and enjoying the day. The mind is alive and focused, and physical tasks don't drain energy reserves.

Among people with type-2 diabetes, exercise can improve insulin sensitivity, which allows for better management of blood sugar, leading to fewer diabetic complications. Daily exercise results in an improved sleeping pattern.

Traditionally, it is well-known that new neuropathways can be developed, but it has been believed that brain cell growth could not occur in adults. Yet, we now know that isn't the case. Neurogenesis, a process by which new neurons are formed, can occur in certain parts of the adult brain.

Exercise can result in neurogenesis in the hippocampus, which is the brain's memory center and navigational center. There is a chemical in the brain called *brain-derived neurotrophic factor* (BDNF) that is used for neurogenesis as a growth factor for these new brain cells. Exercise can increase this growth factor, and the more intense the exercise, the more the neurotrophic factor is increased, up to a certain level. Therefore, exercise has the ability to improve memory.

So what type of exercise is helpful for creating energy? This depends on whether someone is sedentary or exercises on a regular basis. Walking is probably the best exercise for a sedentary person. It can be something as simple and enjoyable as a 20-minute walk around a neighborhood or a walk in a park. The goal is increased energy for the day.

If an increased fitness level becomes a goal, this can be accomplished through gradual progression in exercise. Avoid too much too soon: jumping into an exercise program that is too intense or complex can cause frustration, injury, and exhaustion. Instead, go slow, and know that the body will improve with each session. Duration, complexity, and intensity can be increased over time.

It's useful to develop a habit of going to the gym. Just start going every day, and, at first, do minimal exercise. The gym is a good place and a nice environment with enjoyable people and friends. Eventually you condition your subconscious mind to think of going to the gym every day as a positive experience, a daily reward to look forward to. Soon, it will become a habit and you will be exercising at the gym with friends doing all types of activities.

Maintaining lean muscle mass is essential for healthy muscles needed for posture, lifting, and climbing. It's also important to combine muscle-strengthening exercises at least twice per week to prevent loss of lean muscle mass due to aging.

How much time should you spend on exercise? Twenty minutes five days a week is minimal. I prefer one hour of continuous exercise every day, although not more than one hour. In terms of gaining energy, diminishing returns will occur after one hour of strenuous exercise.

What time of day is best for exercising? Anytime is good, but different times of day each have their advantages. Exercising in the morning provides optimal consistency because it can be incorporated into your morning routine. It raises metabolism, creates energy for the day, and improves mental alertness. In addition, the default waking mental state after a night's sleep is often negative, which can be carried throughout the day; exercising in the morning will disrupt this type of thinking and provide a positive base.

If you exercise at midday, you have a higher body temperature and higher hormone levels, which can help regulate your lunchtime calorie intake. It also relieves stress and gives you energy for the afternoon. An afternoon workout might be best for improving performance and building muscle due to the increase in hormones.

A nighttime workout relieves stress and limits snacking after dinner.

As your exercise program becomes more complex, form is fundamental, but it's even important when you go for a walk or a hike – hunched-over shoulders or shuffling your feet along creates muscle memory that can result in neck pain, low-back pain, and misaligned muscle structures. Walking tall with a straight back builds muscles in optimal alignment.

Posture is paramount. In our society, people simply sit too much, at a desk working on a computer or watching television. Almost always, this posture is with the back stretched out and the chin down or head slumped, positions that have devastating results on the musculoskeletal system.

This is where a personal trainer can be helpful. Certified trainers are educated in proper form and postural deviations. Improved posture results in increased energy because poor posture makes many movements inefficient and painful. Poor posture can cause joints to move improperly. When joints don't function properly, life becomes exhausting and exercise becomes daunting. However, many exercises performed correctly will improve posture, and healthy posture produces energy.

Children and young adults in our society have grown up with video games and computers, and even young athletes now have postural deviations consistent with an older population. They develop "tech neck" from having the head and neck lower than a computer screen. Doctors and dentists develop the hunched back and sore neck syndrome as they lean over patients, the operating table, or the dental chair throughout the day.

There are specialized "posture muscles," and specific posture exercises are needed to keep these strong. One of these muscles is called the erector spinae located from the lower back region to the neck along both sides of the spine. These are underneath the two big power muscles for lifting on each side called the latissimus dorsi (lats). You do not want to use the lats for standing and walking posture. These are so strong they will bring your shoulders and neck down in a stooped, weak-appearing posture. To exercise the spinae muscles, these power lats have to be taken off line. Performing stretching and weight exercises with arms extended above the head will disengage these big power muscles and allow strengthening of the spinae muscles for improved posture.

If you want to increase the strength of the lats, which are used for lifting, you need to perform an opposite group of exercises. For all types of exercise, it's important to learn the right type of exercise for the right purpose.

Form is extremely important for muscle-strengthening exercises. Specific exercises are designed to develop specific muscle groups. If an exercise is not learned and done properly, it can result in muscle pulls and ligament injuries. It's therefore important to learn proper movement patterns and rhythms. Proper form can be used to fix problems, prevent new problems, and ensure maximum benefit from an exercise.

Where should you exercise? Three of the most common options are at home, outdoors, or in a commercial facility. Working out at home is easy but you have the disadvantage of being alone, so you miss out on the socialization and safety aspects of working out with other people.

Exercise outside is phenomenal when the weather is good, the allergy index is low, and the air quality is high. Exercising in nature has been shown to result in twice as much improvement in mood than exercising indoors. Outdoor exercising results in greater decreases in tension, confusion, anger, and depression. Even five minutes of exercise in green space can improve mood and confidence.

Exercising, working out, or doing yoga outside, or playing an outdoor sport, adds a special feeling of experiencing life at a deeper level. It's subtle but once you recognize it, a warm feeling of well-being comes over you. It's especially noticeable when you participate in outside winter sports such as hiking, skiing, or skating on an outdoor rink.

There is not a single word for this feeling in English. The Norwegian language has a meaningful word for this feeling: *friluftsliv*. It was coined in 1859 and has come to represent Norway's allure with nature. The spirit of *friluftsliv* lives inside all of us. The word means walking and climbing in mountains for good tidings. *Friluftsliv* means living in tune with nature, returning to natural surroundings that provide balance and healing.

Some of the top places to run are along the Charles River in Boston, in Central Park in New York City, along Lake Michigan in Chicago, and along the Salzach River in Salzburg, Austria. The people are interesting, the air is clean, there is always something to look at on a seasonal basis, and the scenery is spectacular. Taking a yoga class or other exercise class on the beach is wonderful; try it during your next coastal visit or vacation. Breaking a sweat outside is a good thing. It keeps you alert – that's how our ancient ancestors survived every day.

Working out at a commercial facility has big advantages. You can make it convenient and a routine because there are so many locations. The main advantage of working out at a facility is the social aspect of having friends there, and the variety of exercise options, from free weights and machines to yoga and spinning classes.

Should you work out alone, with a partner, or a group? This is based on personal preference and personality type. Each one has advantages.

Some people like to work out alone because they value their solitary time and set personal goals and challenges for each session.

It's great to have a training partner for one or two workouts a week for safety reasons, such as spotting for lifting, and also for encouragement. A synergy develops with a good partner, which helps you push beyond what you would do on your own.

The group setting for many people is energizing. Spinning, boot camps, and aerobics are great for motivation and camaraderie.

Is walking at work or doing physically active work at the job the same as exercising when you're not at work? Yes, compared to someone who does nothing. Walking and physical activity at work improves a person's mood and energy level. Although for most jobs today, it's not a substitute for a regular exercise program.

A walk in the morning, outside, with a friend seems to put it all together, resulting in the greatest enjoyment and benefit.

———

It was a beautiful early fall morning in New England when I was doing a New York City training run along the phenomenal Charles River in Boston. My pleasant thoughts were interrupted with an even more pleasant thought as I saw my future wife coming toward me. My legs on their own volition made the U-turn to run beside her, and I found myself saying hi to Joan. I didn't get maced, so after some small talk, I asked her for a date, and she accepted. Our first date was at the café above TV's famous *Cheers*, and our second date was the "Halloween Bash" road race, joining 1,000 costumed runners through the streets of Boston.

Our first anniversary saw us running the original marathon from Marathon, Greece, to the Olympic Stadium in Athens. The six-month training for this was magical, especially the 20-mile tune-up runs the three Sundays before the actual marathon. We ran from our Back Bay location to Wellesley and back, except we never seemed to make it all the way back because we would stop for a huge ice cream "mix-in" with all the extras. It was wonderful running together during the tune-up sessions because we drifted into the blissful alpha-brainwave state and the exercise-released endorphins gave us an extra kick of pleasure.

——

Exercise can relieve stress. I had given a seminar in Kyoto, Japan, about the lung disease I described called bronchiolitis obliterans organizing pneumonia (BOOP). Yes, it's a strange name and maybe a funny name for a lung disease, but the acronym was easy for people to remember. However, my scientist colleagues and friends disagreed. "It's confusing and needs to be eliminated!" they shouted at anyone in the meeting willing to listen.

I was devastated. It was a personal attack on my work. After the meeting I felt angry and stressed, thinking *how could the name be eliminated? It would erase all of my efforts.*

So I started running along the Kono River, which was located in the center of Kyoto just like the Charles River in Boston, and kept running toward the mountains. One, two, three miles and my mind was still fuming. During miles four and five, I began to calm down. I was near the base of the hills and turned around to run back to the hotel. The issue began to fade in my mind, and it eventually disappeared completely and had no meaning whatsoever. I couldn't have cared less. It became absolutely meaningless and remains so to this day.

Exercise is a great stress reliever. A small amount of exercise, like going for a walk outside, is needed for typical stress; more prolonged exercise like running, biking, spinning, Zumba, or yoga is needed to help alleviate significant stress. If you exercise enough, your stress will most likely be relieved.

——

The morning started slow for Ed and Sue. They drove to their fitness center for their morning workout. For Ed, it was the spin class. For Sue, it was yoga.

As Ed walked in, guys said, "Hey, Ed, great to see you," before he even got on the bike. The spin class began to fill up with the regulars, and there was a barrage of talk: "How's it going?" "You're looking good," and "How's the 10K training going?" Throughout the spin class, everyone interacted with the instructor exchanging good-hearted barbs. By the end of the class, Ed was going at high energy. This energy level continued in the locker room with the exchange of upbeat comments with another group of friends. After this socializing, he was fired up and more than ready to start the day.

In another part of the workout facility, Sue had joined her yoga group, and her friend had saved her favorite spot for the class. They connected and caught up by talking about their kids. The class began with stretching and challenging body positions, strengthening each muscle group. Sue's friend gave encouragement, which she reciprocated. During the class, the instructor talked about refocusing the mind and dealing with unresolved issues.

Banter among the group of friends continued in the locker room and out the door. The tension that Sue had brought in with her dissipated during the session, and she generated enough energy for an exciting and productive day.

––––

The social part of exercising with a group and at a commercial workout facility such as a gym or studio is unlike any other situation. It's not like connecting with friends at work. It's not like hanging out with friends at a dinner party or cocktail party or a movie or an art opening. Why? Because vigorous physical activity produces those feel-good neurotransmitters, including oxytocin, the human bonding hormone neurotransmitter.

This connection is created with a special group of wonderful friends who come in all different sizes and shapes and include moms and dads, doctors, lawyers, bankers, steelworkers, carpenters, and mechanics – all sharing the common bond of sweat and heavy breathing.

––––

A special section is needed for a discussion for a healthy heart, and people who want to push themselves to their maximal capacity. A vigorous, one-hour workout of pushing 200-pound sleds alternating with 20 push-ups and 20 kettlebell lifts gives a person a great feeling and a tremendous amount of energy. Cyclists in their 40s and 50s can't wait to compete in races and love the feeling of winning – these races take them to sustained heart rates of 160 beats per minute or even higher for hours. They can't stop – they become obsessed with the feeling of competing and winning.

It would be great to work out at that level every week and to compete every week, but no matter how much people want to deny reality, the heart muscle and its electrical system change over time, which becomes a consideration for the senior athlete.

People in their 20s and 30s with healthy hearts can work out and compete with their maximal heart rate without causing harm.

For people in their 40s through 60s and beyond, having a maximal heart rate of 160 to 170 beats per minute for too long can cause an abnormal heart rhythm referred to as *atrial flutter* or *atrial fibrillation*. This in itself may not be a life-threatening abnormal rhythm, but the aberrant rhythm may not return to normal on its own, or even with medication, so an electrical shock with cardioversion in a hospital setting is needed.

Research is underway to further define people at risk and establish a safe heart rate for all ages. In the meantime, keeping a sustained heart rate at a healthy level for your age is a wise decision.

————

Let's check in with Dave and Kate. They're both getting eight hours of sleep a night and have begun to feel increased energy levels.

Leaving her office earlier than usual because of a winter storm, Kate noticed a poster in a shop window announcing that a motivational speaker was giving a seminar about how exercise can change your life.

Hmm, I'm not much for motivational speakers, she thought to herself, but Dave and I don't exercise, so maybe there's something to exercising that can improve our lives. I think I'll go.

Kate went to the convention hall feeling nervous about seeing someone she knew because it would be embarrassing to admit she needed help.

But she quickly found a seat in the back of the room and was soon surprised to discover that she enjoyed what she was learning.

"Dave, we need to start exercising," Kate said excitedly the morning after the seminar. She was motivated! She hadn't told Dave about the seminar because she thought he probably wouldn't have gone, but afterward, she had to tell him.

"What are you saying?" Dave asked, completely uninterested. "The whole world has been telling us to exercise for years, why now? You know I don't like to exercise."

"I really think it could change our lives. It could give us energy."

"Give us energy? It's exhausting!"

"Not really, but fair enough," Kate said, and stopped the discussion for the time being; she didn't want her excitement to be deflated. Instead, she quietly developed a daily exercise program for herself.

Kate had taken some aerobic dance classes in college and remembered enjoying them, so she joined a women's workout facility.

"Welcome, what would you like to do?" Ginny asked.

"Do you have classes?"

"We have about 20 classes during the mornings and evenings," Ginny said enthusiastically. "Which one would you like to take?"

"I'll try the 7:15 aerobics in the morning."

Kate bought some new workout clothes and arrived early to her first session. She found a spot at the back of the class, nervous because she didn't know anyone and didn't want the instructor to criticize her. The instructor flipped on the music from her cell phone, and Kate's nervousness rapidly disappeared. She loved the music and had a great feeling about everyone around her. They were chatting and laughing and seemed to be having a great time.

Kate finished the class and drove to her job with high energy to start the day. She not only had energy, she also felt at peace and stress-free. She soon made the club a part of her life. She attended several different types of classes, including yoga, Zumba, spin, and a barre and sculpt class. She also had wonderful new friends who she looked forward to seeing every day.

"Hi Kate," her new friend, Jennifer said, greeting her with a big hug. "I saved a space for you."

"Thanks. How's your daughter doing in soccer?"

"She's doing phenomenally. She has a game tonight."

"Sounds great," Kate said as the music filled the room and they began their routine.

Several months passed and, suddenly, Dave developed a frightening illness.

"I can't move," Dave said one morning in a concerned, but not panicked voice.

"What's going on?" Kate asked with raised eyebrows.

"My shoulders and back are stiff and painful. Even my hips hurt."

They went to the doctor, and after several diagnostic tests, the doctor told Dave, "You have polymyalgia rheumatica."

"What?" Dave asked, confused.

"The condition is called polymyalgia rheumatica. No one knows what causes it," the doctor said. "It's an inflammatory disease like rheumatoid arthritis, but fortunately it's transient and almost always disappears over time. However, we usually need to treat it with anti-inflammatory steroid medication for several months."

"Sounds complicated," Dave said. "I don't want to take steroids."

"Your concern is understandable," the doctor replied. "This type of steroid is not the muscle-building type; it's the anti-inflammatory type called prednisone."

"I've heard of that," Kate said. "My friend had a bad asthma attack and had to take prednisone. She had a puffy face and gained weight."

"Yes, those are some of the side effects," the doctor said. "We will review them in detail so you can monitor them. Most are reversible, but some can be serious."

"You're right about the reversible part," Kate said. "My friend needed them for a short time. She was completely normal after the prednisone, and after that, she began using a steroid inhaler instead of the pills."

"Dave, I have a tip for you," the doctor said. "You're going to have stiff muscles and pain, and you're not going to feel like doing much, but an exercise program can do wonders for you."

"Exercise? If I'm in pain, isn't exercising the last thing I'll want to do?"

"Maybe, but here's the irony: the polymyalgia will be easier to manage. The exercise will also smooth out the highs and lows of the steroid treatment. Be careful at first, but you should gradually develop a daily exercise program."

"Sounds like I need to do this, but it also sounds like a lot of effort and discipline," Dave said.

"Oh, I know it'll work," Kate said. "Don't worry about the discipline. I'll help you. It becomes such a good part of your day, you'll be upset if you can't make it to a workout."

Dave began his exercise program slowly, just a few minutes every other day. He gradually increased his workout to one hour every day. He joined a workout facility that was on his way to work. He changed up his exercise routine. Sometimes it was the elliptical, sometimes it was light strength training, and he even did a spin class once a week. He stayed at the back of the class so he could go at his own pace, but he enjoyed the camaraderie and support he experienced in the class.

With the help of a physical therapist and trainer, he did exercises that worked around his muscle pain and stiffness. These exercises gave him energy, and as the doctor had said, they smoothed out the highs and lows of the prednisone treatment. The polymyalgia rheumatica lasted for several months but gradually disappeared.

After resolution of his illness, Dave realized that exercise gave him so much energy that he continued to work out every day. He became as enthusiastic as his wife, and they often shared stories about their friends at the club.

When they traveled, Dave and Kate worked out together, going to a spin class or an outdoor exercise class on the beach. These sometimes became a vacation highlight.

This same situation applies to adults who have had a stroke or children with brain injuries, intense and often painful vigorous physical therapy exercise during the first 15 days can result in return to an independent life. If left on their own, these adults and children will go through life with permanent muscular skeletal dysfunction, vulnerable and totally dependent on family and social institutions. Intense physical therapy during the first 15 days is the difference between a life filled creativity and enjoyment or a life filled with uncontrolled dependence on someone else. Exercise can save people's lives.

Your life can change dramatically for the better when you develop a daily exercise routine. It will provide energy, relieve stress, and give you an upbeat feeling to propel you through life with ease and enjoyment.

CHAPTER 11
LEARN SOMETHING NEW
FOR A CREATIVE LIFE

Learn something new every day. Read internet clips, read books, listen to audio CDs in your car, take a class, or find a coach to help you grow and improve. This will give you energy, make you more interesting, make life more enjoyable, and make you more alert. Learning keeps the mind young.

The more obscure the topic and the further away from your work, the better. Consider studying a foreign language and the country's culture or taking a dance class, an economics course, or a philosophy course.

Not many people like to study, and even fewer like to take tests, but everyone likes to learn. New and constant learning can activate and increase energy. Learn something new every day. Just keep learning.

Discovering something new goes straight to the accumbens pleasure center of our brain. Think about how it feels to discover something new. It's a good feeling, a pleasant feeling, a feeling you want to repeat. That's why you keep wanting to learn new things and seek new experiences.

You can make small discoveries like a new route to work, a new food, or a new exotic location. You can also make big discoveries that benefit the lives of people everywhere, a new product, a new device, or a new way of doing things. When you make these big discoveries, you get a bonus – you find enjoyment and pleasure in the process of making these big-impact discoveries.

Learn by searching the internet and watching web videos like TED talks about "ideas worth spreading." You can listen to an entire university CD course while driving, walking, or hiking from companies such as The Great Courses. Learn by doing new things, exploring new places, or experiencing new cultures.

The benefits of learning something new are continually being revealed through research. People who constantly learn have improved health indices, and they have reduced risk of depression. Other benefits include improved well-being and increased self-confidence. Learning engages the brain and creates new neuronetworks. Learning slows the decline of reasoning and memory, and decreases the risk of developing dementia or Alzheimer's disease.

Learning random topics not related to your work or your routine activities can ignite the imagination and create energy. For example, the next several paragraphs are related to arbitrary topics that I have explored.

You can learn how humans learn. Learning occurs from repeated synaptic responses creating pathways in the hippocampus region of the brain. The process occurs through the glutamate neurotransmitter that stimulates long-term potentiation pathways. A second, more powerful two-receptor system has been discovered. This means if enough glutamate is stimulated, it opens a second receptor that floods the receptor with calcium, causing a huge spark of energy and resulting in the pronouncement of "Now I get it!"

There are scores of other subjects you can learn about. For example, you can learn to "think like an economist." These are some of the things you'll learn. People respond to incentives, both positive and negative. Want to discourage people's actions? Add a tax. Want to encourage people's actions? Make the action tax deductible. Pay attention to "opportunity costs" in addition to actual money costs. Consider stress, time lost, gasoline cost, and wear-and-tear cost when driving 20 miles for a five-dollar savings. Whenever there is change – whether it's societal, economic, or work-related – it's always complex and represents many changes taking place. Watch for unanticipated influences and unintended consequences. Pay attention to the margins or fringes of any activity.

You can learn about quantum physics and small subatomic particles that will help you understand strange occurrences that develop in your life.

Genetics has become a major field of study. For example, epigenetics has emerged as a study of the effects of the environment on DNA. The health of the mother and father is reflected in the offspring, which can be carried through several future generations. Pregnancy during a period of starvation will result in illnesses and shorter life expectancy for the offspring from too much methylation of the DNA. Methylation means that one carbon atom and three hydrogen atoms form a methyl molecule, which can become attached to DNA, disrupting the inborn DNA instructions for healthy cell growth and resulting in unhealthy cell reactions such as inflammation.

Epigenetics has shown that babies born of a mother after the mother has gastric bypass surgery have a healthier weight than babies born before the surgery. Another example comes from a study of three generations in Sweden beginning in the 1890s comparing amount of food available and health of offspring. It was found that if food was scarce for the father just before puberty, offspring were less likely to die from heart disease. But if food was too plentiful for the paternal grandfather during the time period just before puberty, death related to diabetes increased in the grandchildren. These examples show that certain types of environmental factors can directly change the DNA.

You can learn about neurotransmitters – chemicals that transmit messages in the brain across two brain cell neurons. Neurotransmitters are stored in packets at the end of the neuron and change a chemical signal into an electrical signal by a corresponding receptor like a lock and key. Some excite the neuron and others inhibit the neuron. There are more than 100 neurotransmitters in the brain and more in other parts of the body.

Too little or too much of a specific neurotransmitter can cause problems. For example, Parkinson's disease occurs from an insufficient amount of dopamine in a specific region of the brain, while schizophrenia results from too much dopamine. So treating Parkinson's with dopamine is effective, but all of the brain receives the extra dopamine, not only the Parkinson's region, so the side effects are schizophrenia-type symptoms. The opposite occurs when treating schizophrenia with anti-dopamine medications.

You can learn about money. Although not equally distributed, money is abundant. Making money does not mean taking it away from someone else. An unlimited amount of money is available to everyone. It's not a game of win or lose. Money can be made without depriving others.

Some people are taught as children that there are two types of people: those with good jobs that improve others' lives through service, and those who are rich. It's either one or the other; you can't be both. And being rich is bad. This limiting belief has frustrated talented and dedicated people and kept them from accomplishing work that was potentially highly beneficial to society. People who are rich can have unlimited compassion and a huge heart to match their bank accounts. Having money to do something good for people or improve people's lives is a good thing, and having more money results in even more good things happening.

"Money is the root of all evil" is a saying that has been shortened over time from the original, which is that "the 'love of' money is the root of all evil." However, money itself is neutral. It's not good or bad. It's what people do with money that creates harm or benefit.

Learn about other random topics. Read about successful people. For example, learn about John Mackey, the founder of Whole Foods Market, and the perspective he developed of American capitalism, which includes providing motivation for people to want to work for a company. In the past, it's been taught the purpose of a company is to maximize profits for shareholders. Not so for John Mackey, who is of the opinion that people don't want to work to increase the wealth of shareholders. His view is that a company needs to have a purpose, and that people want to know that the work they're doing is contributing to helping others and making the world a better place. He thinks a company's decisions need to be made based on the interests of not just the shareholders, but also the employees, customers, suppliers, community, and environment. He feels that a company can thrive at the same time as being socially responsible.

People can learn a better way of doing something, even after 25 to 50 years of doing something the same way. For example, how do you park your car in a parking lot when there are several lines of parking spaces available? Do you pull into the front lane of two-lane parking spots so that when you return, you back out? There's an easier and safer way. If available, drive past the first parking spot into the spot where your car is pointing outward. When you return, simply drive forward out of that parking spot. Then you won't have to strain your neck by looking around several times to avoid cars, people, and animals, nor will you have to worry about hitting another car or a person because you can't see them, nor will you have to worry about someone backing into you because they didn't see you. Try it. It's easier, safer, healthier, and less stressful.

Learn about our English language vocabulary. Why? You'll be surprised. You'll be smarter. The entertaining Professor Kevin Flanigan, who calls himself a "word nerd," brings words to life not only by talking about their meaning, but also about where they came from and how to use them – and often including colorful anecdotal stories about them.

Why are those cheeky silent letters in English words? Because words don't work without them. The g is in the word "sign" because of *signature* and *signal*. The a is in "health" because of *heal* and *healer*. The b is in "crumb" because a cookie *crumbles*. The n is in "column" because a *columnist* writes.

Learn roots of words to learn the meaning of hundreds of words. *Acro* is "height" as in *acrobat* and *acrophobia*. *Log* means "word" as in *logical*. *Pan* means "all" as in *panacea* and *pandemic*. *Phil* means "love" as in *philanthropic* and *philharmonic*. *Junct* means "to join" as in *conjunction*.

Learn to recognize that apparent synonyms may have subtle distinctions in meaning. *Prosaic* means dull in imagination (a prosaic essay); *insipid* can also mean lacking in qualities that interest or stimulate, but its more common meaning is dull in taste (an insipid cup of coffee).

There are just the right words or *le mot juste* for certain situations:

- TV hosts may develop the habit of *vapid* talk, falling flat and uninteresting.
- His friend turned out to be a *perfidious* business partner, turning on him in the end.

- She has a *laconic* style with few words, but always has a quick witty *riposte.*
- Entrepreneurs need to be *Promethean* in their actions – rebelliously creative and innovative.

Sometimes, the best negotiation move is to give someone Hobson's choice – take it or leave it. Take what's available or nothing at all. The stories behind words can be interesting. The origin of the term *Hobson's choice* dates back to the 17th century. Thomas Hobson used horses to carry passengers, packages, and letters between Cambridge and London, England. When he wasn't using the horses, he rented them out to university students. To prevent the horses from being overworked, he rotated them and told customers that they could take the horse closest to the stable door or none at all.

Gap words occur in all languages. There are no words (a gap) for describing certain events and feelings. For example, the English language doesn't have a word for the vapory mist we produce when we exhale below 32 degrees Fahrenheit. We don't have a word for the feeling of being outside surrounded by greenery and fresh air. What do we do about gap words? We make new ones and eventually they catch on and become commonly used. The other way is to borrow them from other languages. Two examples include *schadenfreude,* which means "damage" and "joy" which translates into the feeling of joy when someone else loses, and *weltschmerz,* which means "world" and "pain" which translates into the feeling of sadness from world tragedies. My favorite is *friluftsliv,* the Norwegian word coined in 1859 that translates into English as the positive and uplifting feeling created by several minutes to hours of being outside surrounded by natural green surroundings or wintery surroundings.

Learn about blockchain technology and cryptocurrency. You'll find out that blockchain is computer software that uses "blocks" of information in a "chain." There are three elements of the information going into the blocks. It's global from all around the world. This information is cryptographic, which means hidden coded data that must be unlocked with a digital key. Most importantly, the information going into the chain of blocks is immutable – it's permanent and cannot be changed.

This results in improved businesses and governments by eliminating redundant and inefficient intermediary steps for consumers purchasing goods and services.

Cryptocurrency is digital money and represents a new asset class. The term *crypto* is derived from blockchain technology, which is the underlying technology needed for creation of this currency. More than 5,000 years ago, people were paid with wheat for repairing a house, a barter system. Then, 3,000 years ago, gold and silver coins were created as an asset that could purchase goods and services. In the mid-1800s, fiat currency was established by government "fiat" (order) declaring designated values to a piece of paper money. Now, cryptocurrency has been created as digital money and its value will be determined by members of the global blockchain. Bitcoin created by the original blockchain was the first of many cryptocoins.

Learning something new may result in discovering something you enjoy. Any topic, a musical instrument, a sport, or a job. What about swimming? Pay a small amount of money for a coach. Learn the freestyle stroke and you might love it. You might find yourself looking forward to swimming laps twice a week and your morning ocean swim. You might even do a triathlon. Once you learn how to do something well, you will enjoy it.

Science has shown that finding an expert in the field is the best way to learn something new. When we learn something on our own, we quickly learn what elements and information is needed to learn the skill, and we get good with hours of practice, resulting in a good feeling. We're good at it, but not an expert and not a master of the skill. If you can attain mastery, you will experience the best feeling ever.

It's almost impossible to master something unless you learn from an expert, and it's best to learn from an expert the very first time you do something. This is because when you first learn, your mind is open and flexible, you absorb all the information available to you and find things that work. As time goes on, however, you become more rigid and many of these actions become automatic – completed by the subconscious mind. And, although these actions are good, they may not be good enough to attain mastery without learning from an expert.

For example, you want to learn how to bird-watch, so you begin to observe the colors, the shape of the beak, and the song, and after many repetitions, you get very good, but the experts are so much better. Why? Because they first observe flock behavior and interaction, then they go to the color and song. The same is true for learning sports such as golf, swimming, and running. It's true for learning all new things. Learn from an expert to achieve mastery.

This is a story about learning, memory, and the internet. Students are now being criticized because they can't spell and don't know facts for tests. "It's because of the bad influence of the internet," critics say. This may be true about some students, but it's not necessarily a bad thing. And, these critics may soon find themselves behind times.

Our brain has a limited amount of space for memory. There are two things that fill this space, facts and a retrieval system to find the facts. This is why advertisements that have a product associated with an easy memory retrieval system are successful.

In the past, we used up much of this space with facts. For example, a hundred years ago, people learned Latin and Greek and memorized poems. Then easier retrieval systems became available at libraries so less facts had to be known and a new retrieval system had to be learned.

Now, the internet has almost every fact about every topic in the world. So learning facts is not needed and takes up valuable brain memory space. This newly available memory space is used to remember how to retrieve facts, and people who have learned how to retrieve facts better than anyone else are more successful than people who continue to fill their memories with facts.

Not knowing facts is not necessarily wrong. They're all available on the internet. Learning how to use the new freed-up memory space for retrieving the right facts at the right time and wisely applying them will lead to success.

———

Let's check in on Dave and Kate.

"Kate, I have to tell you what I learned," Dave said excitedly.

"What's that?"

"It's called remote viewing," Dave said.

"Remote what?"

"It's a way of using the mind with your eyes closed to see, taste, smell, and feel things in the past."

"Sounds crazy," Kate said.

"It's a little strange, but it's interesting, and I enjoyed it," Dave said. "You can actually visualize events with your mind, like an oil-field fire and even smell the burning oil. You can see ancient buildings."

"How does it work?" Kate asked.

"Universal energy is like a hologram. Each particle of a hologram contains the whole image. Quantum physics states that each energy particle in the universe contains the past, present, and future. You just need to tune in."

"Sounds like science fiction," Kate said skeptically. "How do you know it's true?"

"You've had an experience when you were randomly thinking about your college roommate 20 or 30 years later, when suddenly the phone rings, and it's your college roommate. How does this happen? Statistical variation or through universal energy?"

"How did you learn remote viewing?" Kate asked.

"I listened to a course in the car while going to work, and with my earphones for some of the exercises because you can't drive while you're doing them. There's a five-day course that's also offered periodically throughout the year. We should go sometime."

"Hmm, a little too strange for me, but maybe."

"There's no harm, and it's a learning experience without any downside, except being embarrassed because you can't believe you will actually see a remote event with your mind," Dave said.

Kate and Dave attended the next class, and found it was an interesting experience, and the alpha brain waves needed to perform the activity filled them with energy.

Next, it was Kate's turn to suggest a new learning experience. "Let's take dancing lessons," she said to Dave one evening after work.

"Hold it. I've gone along with all of these things about sleep, exercise, and the right foods, but I can't go dancing."

"Why not?"

"I don't want to dance with a stranger."

"We can take private lessons, so it's just you and me."

"OK, sounds good, let's go."

Kate signed them up for a weekly lesson. Dave didn't have to worry about changing partners and dancing with strangers.

"That was great," Dave said after the fifth lesson, "and practicing at home was enjoyable. Dancing together produces a lot of energy, and we fall in love again."

"Yup, it's enjoyable, and I liked flying around the dance floor with you and learning the moves."

————

Learn something new? Apply flow conditions. Remember that if you do anything well, you will enjoy it. The more work you put into it, the more you will enjoy it. Adjust your skills to meet the challenge so that you will always know the next step and focus on the task without distractions.

Apply these flow conditions to everything you do during the day, such as brushing your teeth, cleaning the stove, or running errands. The feeling of health and clean teeth. The end result of a clean stove. Meeting friends and interesting people when you run errands. Think about positive events during these mundane activities. You can turn these events into an occasion of flow, resulting in enjoying the day.

Learning to enjoy these activities leads to where you want to go – on to more complex and satisfying creative activities. Increasing the complexity of activities allows the enjoyment of the day to continue. That's why it's helpful to become involved in endlessly complex domains like music, gardening, science, philosophy, and even personal relationships.

Learn something new. You'll be rewarded with unlimited energy and creativity. You might learn something that will help someone else or even your cultural society. Always keep learning.

CHAPTER 12
ALPHA-BRAINWAVE
MEDITATION TIME

Engage in alpha-brainwave time every day. What's alpha-brainwave time? Day dreaming. Meditation.

There are several types of brainwaves based on frequency of the wave. Beta-brainwave activity at 14 cycles per second occurs during our typical waking day. Alpha brainwaves at ten cycles per second occur during light sleep, rapid-eye movement sleep (REM) sleep, and during dreams. Theta brainwaves at seven cycles per second occur during deeper sleep. Slow delta brainwaves at four cycles per second occur during very deep sleep, and 15 minutes of delta-brainwave sleep is required to sustain life. Newly discovered gamma waves are fast and may occur during peak performance.

As an aside, "O" waves, or orienting brainwaves, occur when we go from one location to another. If you have ever gotten up to get something in another room and when you arrived you had forgotten what it was, you've been zapped by the "O" waves.

Learning to be in the alpha-brainwave state while awake will result in many benefits, either by traditional sitting meditation with eyes closed or with eyes open, as I prefer.

You've experienced these alpha brainwaves while you're awake and may not have realized it. These brainwaves will give you a calm, soothing feeling. You may experience them while hiking in the mountains, during a slow jog, shoveling snow, raking leaves on a cool fall day, or even having an enjoyable conversation.

The alpha-brainwave state is being intensely studied, and there are at least five benefits. First, alpha-brainwave time decreases stress by lowering your blood adrenaline levels. You go from the flight-or-fight state to the stay-and-play state.

Second, meditation releases feel-good neurotransmitters and hormones, including endorphin, dopamine, and serotonin.

Third, meditation balances the several realms of your brain – shutting down the rigid analytical temporal lobe, quieting the amygdala anger center, and increasing the accumbens pleasure center.

Fourth, outside activities will give people pleasure and enjoyment, but this is an inside job – meditation brings that pleasure inside with no need for outside forces.

Finally, science-based benefits include improved positive social interactions because of strengthening mirror-neuron function. Mirror neurons are brain cells that enable us to "mirror" people's actions and body language by copying their actions. Mirror neurons help us understand and empathize with each other.

The science of meditation also includes increased telomerase activity. Telomerase is the enzyme responsible for rebuilding the ends of the telomeres, which naturally decline with age. Every cell in our body is constantly being replaced. The telomeres are the protective ends of the chromosomes, but they become shorter with each cell division and eventually become so short, the cell dies. A healthy amount of telomerase will prevent this shortening and prolong cell life, and alpha-brainwave time can increase the availability of telomerase.

Theta-brainwave time can do all of these things and more, especially with improved healing. Learn to experience the alpha-brainwave and theta-brainwave state while awake and experience relaxation, creativity, feeling good, healing, and a new adventure with the mind.

How? The traditional way is with meditation. My way is eyes-open meditation during a walk, yoga, hike, bike, or treadmill run. For example, with eyes open, the Norwegian term *friluftsliv* is used to describe the alpha-brainwave feeling a person develops when outside in free air.

Visual-guided meditation can be an effective method of experiencing alpha- brainwave time and theta-brainwave time. Here's how it works. With your mind, eyes open or closed, visualize a scene and explore the surroundings, stopping intermittently for reflection time.

Let's look at three guided visualizations. The first is for increased personal energy and alpha healing, helping others, and thinking about the past, present, and future by visualizing the empty space of atoms. The second one is for improving speed in your life by visualizing the empty space of the universe. The third is a visual journey along the beach or a mountain meadow for theta healing, theta business, and the joy of feeling good about yourself.

Let's try the first one. In your mind, focus your attention on your hand and visualize the healthy, vibrant cells. Then visualize the nucleus of the cells, then the molecules, and then the atoms of these cells. Now, there is wide and empty space. At the level of the atom, feel the power of the nucleus on your left and the energy of the electrons flying at the speed of light on your right. Put yourself in between the blazing power of the nucleus and the swirling energy of the electrons.

You are surrounded by subatomic packets or particles of pure energy, which I refer to as Level-10 Energy. While you hover in this space, do three things, each lasting one to two minutes.

Breathe in the energy and use the energy wherever needed in the body; and breathe in Level-10 energy sending where needed. After this, think about who you're going to help today – your friend, your spouse, your kids, your coworker, and often times, yourself. After several more seconds, visualize events in the past such as during the last few centuries or even during ancient times. Visualize the life during these times, the day's activities, celebrations or successes. Now visualize your life today. After this, visualize the future – the next few weeks, few years or even the next century. Now, think about the past, present, and future all at the same time, and feel the absence of time. This will lessen the importance of time as causing stress in your life.

A second self-guided visualization takes you from the molecular world of energy to the energy in the spaces of the universe. This time, with your mind, feel yourself hovering above your current location and looking down. Visualize yourself as an eagle flying in the sky. Observe the top of your house and your neighborhood. Fly higher and observe your town or city, your state, and go above the planet and see the green lands and blue oceans of the globe. Then fly beyond the earth and peer at the solar system with the sun and the planets. Now out to the Milky Way.

Keep going and visualize yourself halfway between the Milky Way and the end of the expanding universe. Think of yourself as sitting in a chair and traveling at the speed of the expanding universe. This is fast, more than 42 miles per second. Feel your hair flying in the roar of the speed and feel the wind of pure energy in your face. Feel the speed. This will increase your energy for creativity and accomplishments without stress.

For the third visualization, let's develop your own guided visualization for theta healing, theta business, and a feel-good experience.

Pick an environment such as a beach, mountain, or local park where you begin at ground level and descend 25 wooden steps a beach or meadow.

For example, visualize yourself walking along a path surrounded by tall beach grass waving in a warm breeze on the top of a dune at the beach. As you walk, you cross a wooden bridge over a pond with orange, white, and red koi swimming in the water underneath. Spend time gazing at them swimming softly in the water. You continue your journey along the path until you reach the top of the wooden stairs leading down to the beach and water's edge.

You begin to slowly and quietly walk down the steps, holding on to the wooden railing on the side. Starting with 25 at the top step, you count to yourself the steps down, 24, 23, 22. As you count down, you feel more relaxed with each step, 20, 15, 10. Now you hear the waves quietly landing on the beach, 5, 4. You smell the salty air as you are near the ocean edge, and totally relaxed. It's a beautiful day, warm with a gentle breeze, 3, 2, 1. You step on the warm sand with your bare feet and feel the warm sensation of the soft sand between your toes.

Slightly off to the left you see a canopy with flowing silk drapes hanging from the wooden top and inside, there is a big, soft chair that welcomes you to sit. Then you breathe in theta healing to the specific organ system that needs attention and needs healing. You send healing energy for the healthy cells to replace the dysfunctional cells. You send theta energy to repair DNA and dormant genes that need to be ignited to restore health.

Now you walk toward the right, parallel to the beach where there is a deep blue, bottomless pond. This is a grounding phase. You gaze into the middle of the pond and visualize yourself going through the earth entering the other side, going around the earth and rising up to the top of Mount Everest, and then returning to where you are.

Now that you are grounded in the real world, this is theta-business time. Think about your next step of today's activities, of developing a new idea or a new product, working on a community project, funding a new venture, or starting a business. Think of the next three steps you are going to do today. Give yourself as much time as you wish.

Your final visualization begins with walking to your right toward an ancient wooden door, called the *delta door,* after delta brainwaves. You walk toward the door with your hand outstretched to the ancient wooden handle to open it.

The door disappears as you walk into a golden pavilion with marble tiles on the floor and a fountain in the middle. With your mind, you walk toward the fountain and you begin to notice people all around you. They are warm and friendly and want to see you and talk to you. You are standing near the fountain, your head up. You are filled with strength, gratitude, and compassion. You are filled with success. You are filled with love and grace. People want to be with you and surround you. And, you want to be with them. They want to help you. Talk with them, enjoy their presence because you are the greatest person in the world. Spend time here.

It's time to leave. As you walk away, count yourself down from 5, 4, 3, 2, 1 – returning to the beta-brainwave state of life feeling good, full of energy and excited to see what the day is going to bring you.

You can use this visualization journey with your friend or spouse, visualizing two chairs for theta healing and sharing your time together in the golden pavilion.

The second scene for your own visualization can begin in the mountains or anywhere you wish. You can walk on a mountain path that meanders along a mountainside and opens into a plateau. As you walk along the path you visualize with your mind the different types of trees and shrubs and flowers. You keep walking until you come across an ancient wooden stairway leading you to a green meadow below. You begin counting from the top step at 25 and to 24, 23, 22 … 3, 2, 1, putting your bare feet in the soft green grass of the meadow.

You visualize the different colors of the meadow flowers, the reds, the yellows, the blues, and magenta. The air is warm with a slight breeze as you sit in the soft welcoming chair underneath the silken canopy for theta healing. You walk to your right for the deep blue pond for grounding and consider your next three theta-business action items. You finish your journey walking to your right to the ancient wooden delta door and walking into the golden pavilion, where you are surrounded with wonderful people, and you are filled with success, compassion, forgiveness, gratitude, and love. You count yourself down, 5, 4, 3, 2, 1, back to the beta-brainwave world of pleasure and adventure.

These guided meditations can be used for healing, speeding up your life, business, feeling good, and creating your own use for whatever you need. You can meditate every day for 15 to 20 minutes anywhere you wish at any time. You can join your spouse or friend along the same journey and create a healing place that you can return to when needed.

How do you know when you're in the alpha-brainwave state? Our five senses are governed by our waking beta brainwaves. In the alpha-brainwave state these senses are lessened and perceived differently. You will see a faint fluorescent bluish hue surrounding your head if you're gazing into a bland TV monitor or surrounding the tops of the trees when you're running or hiking outside. It's the same image that you visualize if you stare at a red circle on a white piece of paper for 30 seconds and then look to the side of the circle. The bluish circle you see is the same aura surrounding your face, the trees, or other objects that you see while in the alpha-brainwave state.

Your other senses are also affected. Your hearing is impaired, your sense of smell and taste are diminished, and you have less feeling in your kinetic touch.

How do you know when you're in the deep theta-brainwave state? The blue aura is replaced with a pleasant darkness. Your face becomes featureless in a soft way. You hear nothing. Taste and smell are absent. You have no feeling in your body, your arms, or your legs.

You can use meditation and breathing to increase your personal energy. The body is made up of cycles of energy, and use your breathing to join these cycles. Here's the short version of how to do it.

You can use traditional eyes-closed meditation or eyes open. As you breathe in, use your mind to bring in energy from the bottom of your spine to the top of your head, and as you breathe out, complete the loop by breathing out energy back to the bottom of the spine. Continue breathing in energy from the bottom of the spine to the top of the head and breathing out energy from the top of the head back to the bottom of the spine, making a continuous oval loop of energy.

Move your attention to your chest. Using your mind, breathe in energy through an imaginary opening in the center of your chest and breathe out, forming a cycle of energy. Continue to breathe, bringing in more energy with each breath.

Next, focus on the bottom of your feet. Using the mind, bring in energy through an imaginary opening in the bottom of both feet, and bring the energy throughout the body all the way to your head and then back down again, breathing out through your feet.

The last cycle is with your hands. Using your mind, first pay attention to the energy in the palm of your right hand; then move the energy to the palm of your left hand. You can feel the sensation. Repeat this once. Then breathe in energy through the palms of your outstretched hands, making a cycle through your arms and chest and returning the energy to your hands. Breathe in more energy with each breath. Your hands will tingle with the energy.

Since this is a mind exercise, you'll improve with practice. You'll be able to generate a vast amount of energy.

As mentioned above, you can do this while sitting in a chair or on a pile of pillows with eyes closed, but you can also practice with your eyes open, during a walk or hike, which provides the added benefit of exercise. You can also do this while you're going for a light run, swimming, cross-country skiing, or doing just about anything. Take some time to learn more about the process of focused breathing and energy generation.

Use breathing meditation to reduce stress. Breathe silently in and out, without holding your breath at the top or the bottom of the breath. Breathe equally in and out, and move your lower abdomen out as you inhale.

You can also do yoga "square" breathing, which means breathe in counting slowly to five or ten, hold your breath for the same count, breathe out slowly for the same count, and finish the square by holding your breath for the count of five or ten. You can visualize drawing a square while you're doing this exercise.

After you've stabilized your breathing, you can relax your muscles and release the tension in all your muscle groups. Using your mind, focus on relaxing one area, releasing the tension. Begin with your eyelids, your eyes, your face, the top and back of your head. Relax your neck. You are slowly breathing in and out while you're relaxing the muscles. Using your mind, move to your shoulders and relax them, now the middle back, the lower back, and then your chest. Relax your abdomen with a few belly breaths by breathing in and lifting your abdomen. Return your attention to relaxing your upper arms, lower arms, and hands, and finish by relaxing your upper and lower legs and your feet.

As you continue, you're breathing slowly without making a sound. Your muscles are completely relaxed. As you breathe in, visualize a circulating energy loop moving from the bottom of your spine up to the top of your head and returning back down the front of the spine to the bottom of the spine. It's a continuous loop of energy, always moving. As you breathe in, move the energy from the bottom to the top of the spine and say the word "strength" to yourself. As you breathe out, send the energy from the top of your head, down the front of the spine and to the end of the spine, and say "grace." It's a balance of energy, breathing in "strength" and breathing out "grace." Continue this for a few minutes, enjoying the feeling of energy.

Now do the same thing with your chest. As you breathe in, visualize energy coming into your chest and breathing out, sending energy out of the chest, making a continuous loop of energy in and energy out. With each breath, bring in more energy than the previous breath, not by breathing deeper, but by using your mind. With this breathing, say the word "compassion" for yourself with each breath in and "compassion" for everyone else with each breath out. Continue this for several breaths and feel the energy grow throughout your chest.

Now do the same thing for your feet. Visualize bringing energy through the bottom of your feet as if there are openings allowing the energy in. Breathe in energy, feel it move up your legs, filling your body with energy. As you breathe out, you will complete a continuous loop of energy, increasing energy with each breathing cycle.

The hands and arms are the last cycle. Visualize bringing energy into the palms of your hands, up your arms, and into your body. You will soon feel a tingling in the palms of your hands as they become alive with energy and the energy spreads through the body. Do this for as many breaths as you wish.

Once again, return to the energy loop of the spine, breathing in "strength" and breathing out "grace." Conclude the exercise by returning your mind to the frontal brain, and think about the successful, enjoyable, and creative day you're going to have.

With practice, you'll be able to generate energy with your mind whenever you need an immediate boost. And, this is a wonderful way to manage your stress.

———

Let's take another look at Dave and Kate. Dave developed a habit of negative thinking. Instead of seeing opportunities, he saw problems. This tendency allowed him to identify problems before anyone else, but it developed into a major problem itself for Dave. His negative thinking led to depression and people didn't want to be around him anymore.

"Someone at work told me today that I couldn't say three sentences without talking about a problem or something bad about someone at work," Dave said grumpily. "That was harsh."

"You can change your thinking," Kate said.

"What are you talking about?" Dave asked.

"Negative thinking takes over during adult life by negative conditioning," Kate explained. "This doesn't occur in children. They think in positive ways. So, you need to recondition and retrain your mind to generate positive thoughts, or at least stop yourself from dwelling on negative thoughts."

"And before you start defending yourself by saying, 'I can't change,' here's a fact: everyone can change. And change will make a huge difference," Kate said convincingly. "Dave, constantly bombarding yourself with negative thoughts is depressing."

"I recall someone at work telling me something about the neurolinguistic loop," Dave said. "I wonder if this is related to my depressing thinking."

"I think it is," Kate said. "I read something about neurolinguistics. It has to do with the effect of your own words on the brain causing emotional or physical reactions. Negative thinking sets up an unhealthy negative neurolinguistic loop, which means the relentless negative words can actually create a negative neuropathway for depression."

"How do I change?"

"You change by consciously eliminating the first negative thought. Each time a negative thought comes up, stop it and move on. There's no need to replace it with a positive thought – that's too much work. There's no need to replace it with anything. Move on to something else. Think a negative thought? Stop it and move on.

"That's something new," Dave said. "Why does it work?"

"Because one negative thought leads to two, and that leads to a story, Kate explained. "This is what happens when you have one negative thought. You have a second thought, and the third negative thought builds a story. And, this is always a bad story with an ending that causes frustration, depression, anger, and rage. This is the basis for the adage *think about it, say it, act it, and it becomes your character.* Think negative thoughts, use negative talk, act on negative talk, and you become a negative person. Additional traits of this character include complaining, criticizing, blaming others, and making excuses."

"Sounds like you're right," Dave said. "I'll try it."

Over time, Dave practiced being aware of his thinking and stopped the first negative thought before the thinking went to the dreadful story. Seeing the good in all things was also helpful for him. One morning over a healthy weekend brunch, Dave brought up the subject of breathing.

"I just learned something new."

"What?" Kate asked.

"I learned that you can combine using your mind and your breathing for two huge benefits."

"What do you mean?"

"You can create energy and relieve stress."

"I remember learning about how breathing helps with the pain of delivery in our pregnancy class," Kate said, "but, I didn't know you can use breathing to create energy."

"Try it," Dave replied. "Breathe in the energy that surrounds us and create a loop of energy from the bottom of your spine to the top of your head. Breathe in, sending energy from the top of your head to the bottom of your spine. Then breathe out, sending energy from the bottom of your spine to the top of your head."

"That's easy enough."

"You can also say to yourself *strength* while breathing in and *grace* while breathing out," Dave said. "It gives you balance."

"Sounds good. It almost seems too simple to work."

"It takes practice," Dave said. "I did this during a run the other day, and it turned the run into a pleasant experience."

"Can you use breathing to relieve acute stress?" Kate asked.

"It's easy," Dave said. "Use two or three belly breaths. Put your hand over your belly button, breathe in, moving your hand up. That's all there is to it."

"Hmm," Kate said, as she tried it. "It's tricky. It feels like the opposite of normal breathing, but it has a calming effect."

"I like to use it before giving a big presentation," Dave said. "The other soothing effect is equally breathing in and breathing out, without making a sound. Do this for several minutes whenever you're stressed. It's calming."

"Okay," Kate said. "Now it's my turn to share something with you."

"Do you know what alpha brainwaves are?"

"No idea."

"Well, first of all, there are several brainwave patterns based on frequency that include alpha, beta, theta, delta, and gamma."

"Sounds like Greek to me," Dave snickered at his cliché.

"Stay with me," Kate said. "Beta brainwaves occur during the typical day-to-day brain activity, like getting dressed, driving, eating, and working. Gamma brainwaves are fast, 25 to 100 cycles per second with an average of 40 cycles per second. There's a theory that gamma brainwaves occur in athletes when they're 'in the zone' and play above anyone else."

"Is that what's going on when I have one of those great days closing a huge sale without even thinking about it?" Dave asked.

"Maybe. It doesn't happen much, but it's a thrill when it does!" Kate exclaimed. "The other three brainwaves are related to sleep. Two are exceptional because everyone can learn to use them while awake. It should be taught in school."

"What are they?"

"They're the alpha and theta brainwaves," Kate said. "Alpha brainwaves are seven to ten cycles per second and slower than the waking beta brainwaves at 14 cycles per second. They occur during REM sleep, you know, rapid-eye movement sleep when you're dreaming."

"So that's why you say you're dreaming if I wake you up when your eyes are quickly moving back and forth," Dave said. "And that's alpha-brainwave activity?"

"The exciting part is that you can have the alpha-brainwave state while you're awake," said Kate.

"I think that happens when we run together," Dave said. "After two or three miles of running, we're both floating in space talking about pleasant things and in sort of a dreamy state."

"Exactly, that's alpha-brainwave time," Kate said. "It's pleasant and relaxing. Sitting meditation is the traditional way of experiencing alpha brainwaves while awake, and continues to be the best method, and you can even learn to do this with your eyes open while doing low-intensity activities. It's a creative state of mind. You can come up with creative and useful ideas while in this state."

"I had no idea meditation was so powerful," Dave said. "To be honest, I thought it was a waste of time."

"I thought so too," Kate said, "but I was wrong. Not only can you develop life-changing creative ideas, but the prolonged alpha rhythm waking state has health benefits that are continuously being discovered."

"Okay, you've convinced me about the alpha brainwaves," Dave said. "Now what about the theta ones?"

"They're even more interesting," Kate said. "These are slow, like seven cycles per second and occur while you're sound asleep. But recently it's been found that you can also create the theta-brainwave state through deep meditation."

"Yeah?"

"The body has a vast ability to heal itself if we just create an environment for it to happen," Kate said. "The theta waves that occur during sleep may have a healing effect, but the theta-brainwave state while awake has a strong healing effect."

"Wonderful information, Kate," Dave said. "I'm going to try both of them."

"Incidentally, delta brainwaves occur during profoundly deep sleep and are very slow, at about four cycles per second," Kate said. "The key thing about delta brainwaves is that you have to have at least 15 minutes of this deep sleep each night, or else psychological health will deteriorate. Scientists awakened people during this delta brainwave sleep time for several consecutive nights and began seeing psychological changes. We need the deep delta-brainwave sleep time."

CHAPTER 13
COMPASSION FOR
PEACE OF MIND

Have compassion for yourself. Have compassion for others. *Compassion* is a wonderful word. Tibetan monks meditate by repeating this word over and over for hours, months, and years. You can feel their warmth and kindness being in their presence.

Compassion can combat negative emotions in yourself and from outside sources. Compassion means less self-criticism and being truthful, embracing the good and the bad. The nature of our lives is to seek happiness, and compassion and kindness contribute to our happiness and to other people's happiness.

Professor Kristen Neff has developed profound insight into the benefits of self-compassion. Her perspective about confidence is counter to the traditional thought that self-esteem and self-confidence are positive traits that everyone should strive for. Paradoxically, high self-confidence is only helpful when everything is going well and we are feeling good. When things are going badly for us, and we feel angry and depressed, there is no self-confidence.

Self-confidence and self-esteem only work when you are doing well and don't need them. They abandon you when you're down and need them.

What's Kristen's discovery? Compassion. Develop compassion for yourself. This is powerful when you're doing well – you can share your compassion with others, and when you down, it's a good friend, always there. Out with self-confidence and self-esteem, in with self-compassion. Have compassion for yourself – it always works when you hit rock bottom.

We are often our own worst critic and, too often, beat ourselves up because we made a mistake, we didn't get a job, or we had a trivial fit of anger toward our spouse or friends. We would never punish our friends or family the same way we do ourselves.

So why do we do it? Our brain is built to want to help people, and when we fail, we feel threatened, so our adrenalin kicks in with an increased heart rate, aggression, and anger that unfortunately is directed toward ourselves. We attack ourselves and judge ourselves. Both trigger the amygdala anger center. However, when our friends or family fail, we're not threatened and are kind to them. We fail, we're threatened, and we beat ourselves up. There's no one to be kind to us. During these times *compassion can.*

Professor Neff says to treat yourself with kindness and compassion the same way you would treat others in the same situation. Ask yourself, if you had a friend who was going through the same problem, how would you respond? You would treat your friend with warmth, encouragement, and understanding.

Part of creating an environment for healing is having compassion for the injured area or dysfunctional organ system. Do not be angry with your body. The issue is with the injury or the disease, not with your body that has been affected. Have compassion for the organ system.

Willpower is weak. Use compassion. It's strong and won't let you down. Compassion causes release of the feel-good neurotransmitters and hormones that make you feel good about yourself.

Compassion and kindness can be learned. It has helped troubled schools to overcome problems with bullying and has even changed violent prisons into places of sharing and learning.

Have compassion for others by granting forgiveness. Practicing forgiveness is a common trait among people who enjoy life. Dwelling on the person who caused you pain or the institution that wronged you leads to anger and chronic stress – taking hours, weeks, and even years away from an enjoyable, creative life.

Everyone knows that the anger toward a person or an event has no influence over the outcome, and only hurts us. After going through denial, anger, and depression after a toxic situation, forgive as fast as possible to free yourself from blame and excuses. Stop thinking about the situation and eventually the neuropathway will weaken and wither to the point of extinction.

Having compassion for others increases your positive communications in life and improves your relationship with your family, friends, and coworkers. And, having compassion brings you peace of mind.

CHAPTER 14
GRATITUDE

Be grateful. Being grateful creates a wonderful feeling. It instantly makes you feel good. Stressed out? On the verge of panic? Take a couple of belly breaths and think of things in your life to be grateful for. Grateful for being alive. Grateful for your friends and family. Grateful for feeling good. Grateful for where you live. Grateful for your accomplishments. Grateful for who you are. Being grateful makes you a good person and attracts other grateful people into your life.

The benefits of gratitude have been handed down for centuries. Gratitude has been considered an emotion, an attitude, a personality trait, and a coping response. The Latin derivation of the word has to do with grace, graciousness, kindness, and generousness. Gratitude is linked to well-being.

Professors Robert Emmons and Michael McCullough studying gratitude found that a conscious focus on blessings can have emotional and interpersonal benefits. These scientists randomly gave three groups of students taking a psychology course the task of writing down five things that occurred during the week.

For ten weeks, the first group wrote down five things they were grateful for, such as their own determination to learn, being able to attend the university, and the generosity of friends and parents. The second group wrote down five hassles that occurred during the week, such as finding parking, a messy kitchen, depleting finances, and complaints. The third group wrote down five neutral events, such as talking to someone on the phone or choosing clothes to wear.

The results showed significant improvement in well-being and optimism for the future among the first group of students who wrote down items they were grateful for. They had fewer physical symptoms and increased hours of exercise. The complainer group had opposite findings: a decreased sense of well-being and a gloomier outlook for the future.

These researchers found a similar improvement among individuals with neuromuscular disorders who focused on gratitude. They had an improved positive outlook on life, positive feeling about the upcoming week, positive connection with others, and even improved sleep, resulting in feeling more refreshed on waking.

See the good in all things. This one is easy for some people. For others, seeing the good in all things must be learned through practice. When you're faced with a new situation, rather than seeing its negative aspects, pause instead, and search for the good. This will allow you to fully enjoy the situation if it's a positive event, or to move toward finding solutions if it's a problem.

Seeing the good in people, places, and events will trigger the feeling of being grateful not only for yourself, but for everyone around you.

You can make a habit of being grateful on a daily basis, and if you find yourself low on energy, think of things that you're grateful for. It instantly improves your energy and your positive outlook on life.

CHAPTER 15
YOU CAN LEARN
SELF-HEALING

Just as machines are built to repair themselves, you are too. Healing is a state of mind. It's restoring physical health from injury or disease and restoring mental and emotional health. It's using your mind to manage injury and disease.

To begin, learn everything you can about what you're facing. Ask your doctor questions and search the medical educational sites for anatomy of the injury and process of the disease. Learn the diagnostic testing used to confirm the extent of the injury and the correct diagnosis.

Research the best treatment option for your situation. Find out the natural history of the problem which means what happens if no medical intervention is used, which will help you know what to anticipate. Find out the benefits of other options, including antibiotics, medications, or surgery, and the associated risks with each of these options. Choose the one that's best for you. After this, monitor the injury or disease over time with symptoms or objective measurements.

Now, it's time to create an environment for healing through self-healing. Start by using a positive approach. Tell yourself that you can manage the situation. You will not allow the disease to control you.

Approaching the disease in a positive manner will help you avoid the negative neurolinguistic trap, which is caused by repeatedly thinking about and verbalizing negative feelings about the illness. These negative thoughts create a new neuropathway that becomes cemented in your brain, sending you down the road of perpetual aggravation, chronic pain, depression, or even worse.

Next, have compassion for the injured area. It can heal naturally over time. Have compassion for the diseased organ system. The system is functionally healthy. The disease is causing the dysfunction.

Use controlled breathing to create a healing environment. Three methods can be used. Trigger the relaxation reflex with a few belly breaths by deeply breathing in and moving your stomach outward. Breathe with equal breath in and equal breath out for one to two minutes. Use the yoga square breathing by breathing in while counting to ten, holding your breath for a count of ten, breathing out for a count of ten, and holding for a count of ten.

An important part of these breathing exercises is to tell yourself, while you're breathing in deeply, that you're breathing in healing energy and Level-10 Energy for healing. Send this healing energy to the entire body from the top of your head to the end of your fingers and toes. And, send this healing energy to the specific injury site or to the diseased organ.

You have now approached the disease in a positive manner. You have learned everything you can about the disease. You are using controlled breathing methods. Visualization is the final step for creating a healing environment.

Optimally, use visualization while in the alpha- or theta-brainwave state through traditional eyes-closed meditation or my preferred method of eyes-open meditation. You can create a "healing place" in your mind during your alpha-brainwave time, and you visit this place for healing visualizations.

There are several visualizations that you can use, and you can also create your own based on the injury or disease.

First, as you breathe in, send healing energy to the specific body part that needs healing, such as the knee or organ system. The more specific, the better. For example, send healing energy to heart arteries, heart muscle, or the heart electrical system.

Next, with your mind, replace dysfunctional cells beginning with one cell replacing the injured cell. Every cell in the body is continually replaced, some every few minutes and others every few weeks or months.

Visualize healthy, strong cells replacing the inflamed or dysfunctional cells. Replace cells exponentially beginning with two cells, then four, then eight, and eventually replace one million cells using visualization.

Renew the DNA in your cells. You were born with DNA instructions for a healthy functioning body. Over time, methylation of the DNA may cause damage and sluggishness. Renew the DNA alignment with your mind.

Switch on your dormant healing genes. Epigenetics tells us the environment can greatly influence the activity of our genes. Over time, genes that generate certain types of enzymes and reactions in the healing process gradually become switched off. Turn them back on with your mind.

Be persistent, as these methods require repetition and time in terms of weeks, months, and years.

Let me tell you about John. He's an energetic guy who was doing repairs on one of his rental properties when he tripped over a cord and landed on his left shoulder. An MRI showed a tear in the rotator cuff.

Off to surgery for repair? Not John. He explored physical therapy, an excellent choice that is often overlooked as a treatment alternative. During his introductory session of anatomical review and measurements, he talked to a fellow patient who was grimacing in pain from the exercises.

"What'd you have?" John asked his co-inhabitant while his physical therapist was in another room.

"I had rotator cuff surgery two weeks ago," and I'm in for physical therapy.

John confirmed his thinking, if you have to go through this after surgery, why not go through it now? Thus began his grueling sessions. At the beginning, he could not raise his left arm above 90 degrees. That's where his physical therapist started. The pain became so bad during one of the sessions that he had an episode of shock with sweats, chills, and shortness of breath. The sessions were finished with an ice pack to lessen his pain before returning to work.

His orthopedic doctor told him that he had a 50 percent chance of recovery without surgery. The failure rate often occurs in people who give up and quit the physical therapy – too painful, too slow, and too much work.

John had the right approach. He heard the stories about frozen shoulder, about people who had the arm in the 90-degree locked position for their entire lives. He made up his mind that he would do whatever it takes not to have this happen to him. He was not going to have a dysfunctional left arm, and would only settle for a fully functional arm.

John used negative visualization to do this. Every day and night, he visualized his arm being frozen at 90 degrees for the rest of his life, and this was intolerable. Visualization was a powerful motivator for him. He stayed with the physical therapy and emerged six months later with his left shoulder activity back to normal.

Others may use positive visualization by visualizing their arm rising straight above the shoulder at 180 degrees.

Dr. Michael Moskowitz, a pain management specialist, talks about his personal experience with pain in his neuroplasticity transformation book. He injured his neck in a water-skiing accident that led to chronic debilitating pain when he was 45. He used several traditional medications without relief.

So, he tried visualization. He repeatedly visualized shutting down the brain's pain center from firing pain signals. He also forced himself to ignore the pain and concentrate on his writing and work. Distraction is an effective method for pain management. His brain eventually rewired itself to focus on the task and shut out pain signals. His pain diminished in a few months and was gone in two years. The brain has neuroplasticity – it can be rewired by building new neuropathways.

Visualization, distraction, and sounds can rewire the neuropathways away from the pain signals, restoring healthy brain signals from the pleasure center.

Dr. Lissa Rankin talks about self-healing in her book *Mind Over Medicine*. Take advantage of the placebo effect. What's the placebo effect? It's the elimination of disease symptoms by the mind.

Some placebo stories are legend. Giving sugar pills for treatment of disease and finding they are more effective than the medicine. Curing hyperventilation syndrome with a saline injection, a harmless salt solution. Performing a surgical operation by opening and closing, and finding it more effective than performing the complete operation. Studies show that 20 to 30 percent and even higher of all medical treatments are solely from the placebo effect.

Almost everyone has experienced the placebo effect. Think about it, drinking hot water thinking it's tea, and finding out later you didn't even put in the tea bag because you're in love.

There's a dark side to placebos – it's the nocebo effect. Too often, people who believe they have a non-treatable disease develop the nocebo.

For example, in double-blinded studies when people are warned about specific side effects, up to one-quarter of participants receiving the non-drug, innocuous pill will experience these side effects such as vomiting, muscle weakness, colds, or memory loss, and sometimes even more serious side effects. Some may even lose their hair if it's a cancer-treatment study. People who convince themselves they're going to die from a routine surgical procedure and a minor illness often do die.

A person whose father died at age 52 or another specific age thinks about this age throughout life, and this person may die at this exact age. People who are told by their doctors that they have three years to live may die exactly three years later even though they've been cured.

The lesson from these stories means that we have an extraordinary ability to heal ourselves, and the opposite, we can become ill or even worse by concreting negative feedback neuropathways.

Approach the injury or disease in a positive manner continuously at all times. Negative beliefs are destructive.

It's important to associate yourself with the right group of doctors and medical people who are optimistic and supportive. It's especially important to surround yourself with friends who are positive and who don't continuously complain about their ailments. Do not consider your illness incurable or chronic. Believe your condition can be managed. After all, managing your injury or illness is good enough.

Managing chronic stress is part of the healing process. We deal with stress every day. Surprisingly, acute stress doesn't hurt anyone. The human system has evolved over thousands of years to manage acute stress with the appropriate amount of stress-response hormones and neurotransmitters.

The flight-or-fight response caused by a surge in adrenaline results in increased heart rate and blood pressure, as well as shutting down the stomach. In healthy people, the stress response can be triggered by events of day-to-day living, such as an argument, a parking ticket, or a dripping faucet. The response lasts for a few minutes, then dissipates.

The body is well equipped to handle this without harmful effects. Helpful techniques to dissipate this type of stress include a few belly breaths, yoga breathing with equal in and out breathing, and repeating a mantra such as "love and peace" for 45 to 60 seconds.

Chronic stress is a killer. It will cause life-threatening health problems and drain energy. To counteract this, learn about chronic stress and how to manage it. Recognize when you're in a chronic stress situation. Examples include loss of income; being in a work setting with a tyrannical, controlling boss, supervisor, or coworker; living with an alcoholic or drug-using family member; or caring for a spouse or parent with Alzheimer's or another disabling condition.

Chronic stress resets the adrenalin level to a continually higher level, resulting in rapid heart rate, increased blood pressure, shutting down digestion, and causing inflamed arteries.

There are three reasons that we have not adapted well from the acute stresses of the ancient world to our new-world environment of chronic stress.

First, we live in a widely different environment than our prehistoric ancestors. We live in cities, we race through the day in our automobiles, we fly from one city to another in hours, and we are now highly dependent on electronics, cell phones, and computers, all setting us up for the chronic stress of rushing to make deadlines and meetings, competing for space, and unexpected breakdowns and delays.

Second, we almost always experience delayed return in everything we do, and without guarantee of success. We work for hours, weeks, months, and sometimes years doing things that have no immediate return. For example, a farmer plants, waters, does weeding, and harvests all for the future, yet faces the possibility of crop failure at any time. Graduate students work for years not knowing if they will actually get their degree or if they'll find the job of their dreams after earning that degree. We hope for the return of our efforts later, sometimes in a few weeks but often in many years, and this creates chronic, and sometimes severe, life-threatening stress. Counter this by enjoying the process and not the goal.

Third, we feel the need to be in control at all times. In reality, most events are beyond our control. We personally cannot do anything to control the lion's share of situations, but we think we can because of the technology available to us. Striving to be in control at all times creates chronic stress.

The chronic stress response varies widely among people because stress is the physical and emotional response to a person's *interpretation* of an event or threat. Stress is a fear-based reaction. A plane ride with up and down loops is exhilarating for some, producing healthy neurotransmitters and hormones, but terrifying for others, producing stress hormones and toxic chemicals.

There are two parts to the stress response. First is the event and second is the perceived ability to cope with the event. For example, some people put themselves in stressful situations all the time – such as starting a new company or running for public office – because they know they can cope with the circumstances, while others interpret less intense situations – such as going to a social gathering or meeting new people – as stressful because they feel they cannot cope with circumstances.

Coping with stress. Use the five components of well-being and the ten health practices. Learn to focus on what's intrinsically important to you and discard or ignore everything else.

People who are better able to cope with stress are self-compassionate. This means treating yourself with kindness and forgiveness when bad things happen, especially when it's your own fault. Be kind to yourself and forgive yourself.

Use breathing for stress relief. Take a few belly breaths. Use the equal-in and equal-out breathing technique for several minutes. These techniques have a calming effect on the vagal nerve system.

While going through the day, consider the amount of stress related to your daily choices. Choose the less stressful alternative. It may take longer or be less convenient, but the choice will be less stressful and less toxic to your health.

Consider the amount of stress involved in making financial decisions. Take the less stressful option even if it costs more. Pay the additional cost for a product rather than go five miles to buy the product on sale or at a discount store. Pay someone to do work if this is less stressful than doing the work yourself. Even consider the amount of stress required to make the money to pay someone. If making the money is less stressful than paying someone, pay them.

Other examples of choosing less stressful situations include walking behind a stopped car instead of walking in front of the car. Park and walk rather than repeatedly circling the block to find a parking spot close to your destination. Make right turns to avoid stressful left turns. Drive rather than fly for short flights. Consider the amount of stress related to your daily choices. Make the right health choices.

Financial stress can destroy people's lives. This requires a special section because this type of stress is common but often overlooked. Everyone has experienced financial stress for short periods of time or, all too often, for several years.

This type of stress occurs when the amount of money you have coming in is not enough to cover the amount of money that is going out. It's stressful when your paycheck is spent on bills and expenses, and there is none left over for anything else – or worse, when you can't pay all the bills and you have to scramble to find money elsewhere, usually from credit cards or borrowing through debt.

This creates a terrible feeling of despair and source of worry. This may lead to anger, blame, excuses, rationalization, and resentment, all causing stress.

Financial stress is especially dangerous because it occurs on a daily basis and leads to unhealthy results. It interferes with pleasure and can destroy relationships. It's critical to eliminate financial stress from your life.

The solution lies in a simple concept of living with more money coming in than going out, more income than spending, and as debt causes stress, minimizing and eliminating short-term debt is helpful.

How to live with more in than out? Use the power of conditioning the subconscious mind.

Mike Michalowicz discusses a method of eliminating financial stress in his book, *Profit First*. Have separate accounts for profit, savings, and expenses. Add a tax account if you're self-employed. Determine percentages of income that go into each account. When money comes in, deposit it into the profit account first, then the savings, and then the expenses. The first two accounts are separate from your day-to-day checking account for expenses. This is the subconscious mind working – out of sight, out of mind, so you don't spend it or use it to buy things. If the expenses account is too low to pay the bills, review and cut out things you can live without until there is sufficient money in this account to pay living expenses.

If you have short-term credit card debt, use 95 percent of the money in the profit account to pay this off. Then use 50 percent of the money in this account to pay off long-term debt until you have no debt. Then you can spend 100 percent of the money in the profit account as you choose.

The savings account is off limits until it becomes large enough to invest and eventually this will yield an income sufficient to pay your expenses. Then you have arrived at financial independence, and have eliminated financial stress.

Keep Parkinson's Law in mind: you spend what you make. You make ten dollars, you spend ten dollars. You make $50K, you spend $50K. Don't let yourself fall into this trap. You can enjoy your life and do whatever you want. Live frugally, but not cheaply.

There are five rules to help live a frugal lifestyle. First, always look for free options. Second, buy used, especially cars. Third, never pay full price, negotiate. Fourth, delay major purchases until you've reviewed several alternatives. Finally, use the "one more day" or "can't live without it" phrases for any purchase. Considering buying something? Wait one more day. Considering buying something? Ask yourself, "Can I live without this?" The answer will help you make the right financial decision.

Explore fear as a basis for stress. Positive emotions include joy, gratitude, love, pride, and serenity. Negative emotions include fear, anger, sadness, guilt, and shame. Frustration is a combination of emotions. Why do you need to be reminded of these emotions? The easy answer is that positive emotions create energy and eliminate stress, and negative emotions use up energy and produce stress.

It's important to know the meaning of emotions. Sadness means the loss of something, either real or symbolic. Anger is the feeling that something has been taken away, a perceived violation or injustice. Fear means a perceived threat.

Fear is often the root cause of chronic stress. Fear of a controlling boss, fear of losing your job, fear of an abusive spouse or child, and fear of an uncontrollable situation.

You can eliminate stress by realizing that it's being caused by your interpretation of a threat. It's not the fear, it's your reaction to the fear that's causing the stress.

When we eliminate the fear, we eliminate the stress.

Fear and anger are so powerful that they can actually destroy life. Conquering these emotions offers a solution to chronic stress.

Consider two groups of people who are outwardly healthy and who are similar in age, background, and weight. Even though both groups exercise, people in the first group are more at risk for a heart attack than people in the second group. Exercise helps to prevent heart attacks, so why would any of these people have a heart attack?

People in the first group exercise out of fear of having a heart attack. They're angry about being forced to exercise. They trudge through exercise every day and complain the whole time. The second group? They *love* to exercise. They enjoy it. They look forward to how it feels. It creates energy, it improves muscle tone and posture, it activates the feel-good neurotransmitters, and as a bonus, it allows them to see their friends. People in this group are not going to have a heart attack.

People in the first group are doing fear-based exercise. The fear of a heart attack is so great that it produces cortisol and other damaging chemicals that far outweigh the benefits of their way of doing exercise. The solution is to approach your daily exercise in a positive way. Learn to feel the benefits. It could save your life.

Fear-based actions occur in many other areas of our lives, most of the time unknowingly. Here's another example: two groups of people eat the same foods, yet some will develop diabetes, hypertension, and heart disease. Why? They're forcing themselves to eat "healthy foods" and are filled with anger and chronic stress about having to eat foods they don't like. They're trying so hard to eat healthy foods or follow the latest diet that the cortisol and other toxic chemicals produced by these emotions cancel the benefits of healthy eating.

People in the healthy group, however, love to eat healthy foods. They learned how to enjoy the subtle and new tastes of foods with no added sugar, no added salt, and no processed omega-6 fats. They learned to love the taste and texture through positive conditioning, and they enjoy the feeling that the food is not going to harm them. You can condition yourself to enjoy eating healthy foods and savoring the taste.

Another example: two groups of people have the same job, and some people will develop hypertension and heart disease while others thrive. You know the people who are destined for disease. They dread going to work, struggle through the day, and incessantly complain about the job. They're angry about having to work, and yet are in constant fear of not working. They can't wait for five o'clock so they can escape the drudgery that they have created for themselves. This chronic stress, anger, and fear culminate in deadly levels of cortisol release and toxic-reaction chemicals day in and day out, causing chronic inflammatory diseases such as hypertension, heart disease, and even cancer.

People in the second group have spent time and thought into learning to love their jobs. They look forward to going to work. It gives them energy. They enjoy meeting the challenges and talking to people, and they enjoy the workday. Even if they are not naturally experiencing their passion and their life's calling, these people learn to find a way to enjoy their work.

Regardless of what your job is, it can become enjoyable. My friend Marco was in his 20s and worked at a car wash making minimum wage, and he loved it. I saw him there for years. He was always smiling and had a quick, friendly hello and made light, pleasant conversation with the customers. For him, he didn't work at a car wash. He went to a place to talk to people. He loved to see people and speak with them. He was doing his most favorite thing: talking to people.

Over time, Marco started his own car-detailing business and expanded the business to several car-detailing outlets. He's on his way to financial success and a healthy energetic life. He never consciously thought of this while working at the car wash. Because of his positive attitude, opportunities developed, and he had boundless energy. He found enjoyment in his job and success followed.

———

Overcoming fear can save your life. To do so, you must know that the body can heal itself. Ask Buck, who was interviewed on a radio show about his experience.

He is a successful entrepreneur, busy husband, and father of three children. He was training for a triathlon and overdid his gym workout. He built up too much lactic acid from anaerobic metabolism and too much muscle fatigue. He developed a rapid heart rate referred to as atrial flutter, which can happen to people over 40 who push their heart rate past 150.

"Buck, great to see you today, tell us what happened," the interviewer asked.

"My heart rate didn't slow down after my shower, and it kept going at a rate of 135 beats per minute for a couple of hours."

"What'd you do?"

"I went to the ER and the cardiologist brought the rhythm back to my normal rate of 58 with a cardioversion shock while under anesthesia," Buck said nonchalantly.

"You make it sound so trivial, you could've died," the interviewed said in disbelief.

"I didn't think about it. I love to work out, and the heart rate was back to normal," Buck explained.

"What happened next? The interviewer asked.

"At first I denied anything had happened and returned to my training. But then, almost immediately, I became so nervous that I couldn't work out. I began thinking that I would never work out again."

"Why were you so nervous?"

"Fear. I was afraid that if I worked out too much, the out-of-control rapid heart rate would start again. I feared I would have to be shocked again. I feared I would be limited by my heart. I go full-out or not at all. I was afraid my life would be shortened. I became afraid of the future."

"Sounds scary. What happened?"

"I tried working out and had a panic attack with sweats and shortness of breath after my heart rate doubled, which was safe enough, but I didn't know if it was the good rate or the bad rate. Fear gripped me so strongly that I had to stop. It was frustrating and created a vicious cycle of fear by not doing enough exercise, which created more fear, which generated more fear again."

"You were heading for trouble. What'd you do?"

"It took a while, but I realized that fear was the problem, and that I had to eliminate it or go on living at half speed, an unacceptable option."

"What'd you do?"

"I tried an easy solution. Build my confidence back up one day at a time by running a little more, swimming longer, and slowly lifting more weights to prove to myself that my heart could build back up to normal," Buck said.

"Did it work?"

"Not even close," Buck said with a sigh. "The fear continued to cause episodes of extra beats. It was worse than ever."

"What'd you do then?"

"I tried will power, telling myself over and over that I had no fear. That didn't work at all. I kept having skipped heartbeats and had to slow down, which made the situation worse. It wasn't like a broken bone that heals in six weeks and is stronger than ever. This was a heart problem that was only going to recur and get worse. This fear generated a huge outpouring of toxic chemicals, causing all types of problems, especially an increased heart rate."

"You tried the recommended methods, but they failed," the interviewer said, summarizing his attempts to find solutions. "So, what'd you do next?"

"There are always options. I kept exploring them. I learned that the body has an ability to heal itself. I needed to find out how. For me, it was through meditation and using alpha and theta brainwaves along with visualization," Buck explained.

"Please tell me more."

"Theta brainwaves are the slow ones that occur during sleep and have some effect on health while sleeping. By creating the theta-brainwave state while awake through meditation, healing can take place," Buck said.

"That makes sense," the interviewer replied. "Go on."

"Once in the theta state, I focused my attention on the heart muscle, the heart arteries, and the heart electrical system, sending healing energy to these systems. I did this every day for weeks."

"Did you do anything else?"

"I visualized repairing the heart DNA. All of our cells continually renew themselves, and the DNA has built-in repair systems that keep it the same as at birth. So visualizing the repair process will return the DNA to the original state to create a healthy heart cell during the next growth division cycle."

"Did this work?"

"Visualization works for programming muscles for athletic training and may also work for repairing DNA. If nothing else, I was in control by trying to do something."

"Did you do anything else?"

"I also visualized igniting dormant healing genes," Buck said.

"Like repairing DNA, that sounds a little far-fetched," the interviewer said, skeptically.

"It's the same as repairing the DNA. Over time and inactivity, heart-healing genes become dormant. While in the theta brainwave state, visualizing igniting these dormant genes can activate them to create healing proteins."

"You used visualization to send healing energy to the electrical system of the heart, repair heart cell DNA, and activate dormant heart genes. How did this help you?" the interviewer asked.

"It made the fear go away," Buck explained. "I realized that my heart could return to being normal and healthy so the fear vanished. Now it had become like a broken bone; over a six-month period, it would heal and be as strong as before. Therefore, I could continue working out in a 'controlled' manner without fear. The fear-based life was gone."

"I'm pleased to hear this worked for you," the interviewer said in closing.

_____

Let me share a story about Michael. I was a guest on his radio show. He told me he had developed lung cancer, which had spread to his heart. He took the news as anyone would, as a death sentence. He feared the upcoming surgery. He feared that his life was going to be cut short. He feared he would have to leave his family. He feared no longer being able to do his life's work. He feared death. The list of fears went on and on. This is a normal and expected response.

But the normal response stopped there. Somewhere in the back of his mind and for a reason unknown to him, he understood clearly that he wanted to be fit and strong for the lung surgery, so he increased his exercise program. Suddenly, after working up a profuse sweat, his heart pounding, and his breath coming fast, Michael's fear of death vanished. And all the other fears vanished too. He underwent the surgery with profound success. He had no chemotherapy and no radiation. He was cured. That was more than a decade ago. Today he continues to be grateful for every minute of the day and enjoys life to the fullest.

Use the neuropathway bypass technique. If you determine that the cause of your chronic stress is a controlling, abusive boss, coworker, spouse, or someone else in your life, then use the neuropathway bypass technique to permanently eliminate this specific stress.

What is the neuropathway bypass technique? You bypass the negative stressful neuropathway.

When you see this controlling or abusive person, hear the person, or even see the name on a document or cell phone, you instantly develop a knot in your stomach along with increased blood pressure, increased breathing, sweaty palms, and a rapid heart rate. The stress spirals out of control, and if left unchecked will lead to serious illness.

Instead of using this unhealthy, ingrained neuron highway, create a healthier track with a bypass. The method is simple to carry out but does require a short period of discipline. This can be applied to all types of unpleasant situations. It takes two minutes each morning for two weeks.

Here's how it works. In the morning, visualize the image of the feared or aversive person in your mind until it triggers the anger-related feelings in the pit of your stomach. You can do this during your morning routine or during your morning run or walk.

When the feelings of discomfort develop, begin saying two soothing words to yourself repeatedly – "love and peace" or "peace and strength." Say the words over and over until the feeling of anger subsides, usually in about two minutes. The next morning, do the same thing, visualize the angry image in your mind, allow the knot of anger to develop in your stomach, and again repeat the two words to yourself until the unpleasant feeling subsides. Repeat this exercise every morning for two weeks.

Sarah tried it. She had a controlling, abusive boss who was causing unbearable and unhealthy chronic stress. So, during her early-morning run, she triggered the knot in her stomach by visualizing her boss berating her. She started repeating "love and peace" to herself over and over, and found, to her surprise, that in less than two minutes, the feeling completely disappeared and was replaced by a soothing feeling.

However, this calming feeling didn't last long – the minute she saw her boss's car in the parking lot, the anguish quickly returned. This is expected, the aberrant neuropathway had taken months or years to create, and it will take time to build a bypass.

So, on the way home from work, Sarah repeated the exercise. The tightening in her stomach quickly returned as she visualized her boss, but again she was pleasantly surprised to find it was then replaced with a soothing feeling. She continued the exercise for several more days.

Around the seventh day or so, she realized that, when she visualized her boss, she was having a hard time triggering the unpleasant feeling in her stomach. This was strange, and she didn't believe it at first, but after two more days, no matter how hard she tried, she couldn't trigger the fear and anguish when she visualized her boss. It was a wonderful experience.

This new development gave her a renewed feeling of strength. After two weeks, Sarah realized that when she saw her boss or heard the name at work, it meant nothing to her. She had no fear and no stress. Her face appeared serene. She was no longer a victim.

Several days passed, and her boss was about to begin the usual verbal public lashing during one of Sarah's team meetings. She was standing about 12 inches away from her boss's nose. She looked directly at the pupils of her boss's eyes and smiled. At that moment, Sarah had an overwhelming feeling of calmness with no increased heart rate, no anger, and no fear. The boss blinked a couple of times, said nothing, and left the room.

Months of hostility had come to an abrupt end. The boss later found someone else to torment. Sarah returned to her work full of energy and enjoyed her creative work. She was so successful, she soon left this position and moved to a higher-paid and more enjoyable job.

If you find yourself in a "negative-feedback" loop, learn the bypass method. You can use it in multiple situations. As time passes, it will take less than a few days to develop a bypass. You regain your strength. Your creativity returns. You are a stronger person.

Manage workday stress. If you determine that your chronic stress is from your work, then start by managing your mind at work. Stress, anger, and worry top the list of unhealthy feelings. How do you deal with these issues? The single most important factor is to develop a positive approach to your workday, no matter what the conditions are. It's an excellent way to deal with unhealthy feelings, and a bonus is that you'll have more energy and enjoy your work more.

Look for the good in all things. Be grateful. Keep returning to a positive attitude – it's healthy and clears your mind to solve problems and improve the overall situation. Staying positive will help you manage the stress, anger, worry, and interpersonal work relationships, and it can even help manage deadlines.

A common but less known cause of stress at work is moral stress. This comes from working at a company that bends rules and violates rules with deceptive and false advertising and unethical financial manipulations.

Company executives know the consequences of an investigation can destroy the company. However, they allow these practices to happen by justifying to themselves that the company needs to be financially successful to provide jobs. But, underneath this rationalization lies the truth: executives don't think they will get caught.

Unfortunately, this is often true. They don't get caught, but these companies will eventually fail because employees will be miserable and nonproductive. Working in an environment of deception and lies causes tremendous stress. The majority of employees observe the behavior going on around them all day long, and don't say anything because of peer pressure and fear of losing their job.

This moral stress is dangerous to your health and needs to be managed before irreversible health effects result. Review the situation, and consider that leaving for another situation may be a healthy alternative.

Stop the first negative thought as a method of eliminating stress. Each time a negative thought comes up, stop it and move on. No need to replace it with a positive thought – that's too much work. No need to replace it with anything. Move on to something else. Think a negative thought? Stop and move on.

Use this method to manage a series of rejections. You've submitted proposals, loan applications, college applications, or funding plans for a project or startup; and you've received two, five, ten, twenty, or more rejections. We're told that rejections are part of life and part of success. The first few are ignored, but eventually you begin to think about these rejections.

You tell yourself you're a failure, you're not smart enough, and everyone else is better than you. These negative thoughts begin to repeat themselves incessantly until you convince yourself you're a failure at everything, and the world is out to get you. These thoughts go on and on day after day.

You become irritable and depressed. You become angry and rage at your family and friends. You don't want to be around people because you're so upset; likewise, people don't want to be around you because you're negative and depressed. All of this started from a single negative thought.

You've been chewed out at work. You've been fired. You've been turned down for a job. You don't get a promotion. A negative thought about this pops into your head. Do not have a second thought. Do not replay the scene.

You have an illness or an injury? Stop all negative thoughts about these. A parking ticket? You've been criticized? Do not have a second thought and do not replay these scenes in your mind. Distraction is the best way to stop this thinking. Focus on something else.

What happens when you master this technique? When you stop the second negative thought? You have an instant feeling of relief. Your whole body is relieved because you don't have to relive the depressing story again.

Over time, the story will disappear from your memory. You free your mind to be healthy, more creative, and to lead an enjoyable life.

Procrastination as a cause of stress. Here's another cause of stress. It's procrastination.

What to do? First, to get something done, get in motion because once in motion you stay in motion. Do whatever it takes to move, something tiny, say one word, type two words, or move out of the chair. Once in motion you stay in motion. You need to get started, once started you stay started.

Use the brain regions to your advantage to manage procrastination. Doing that small step to get started sends a message of accomplishment to the nucleus accumbens pleasure center. This in turn creates a positive pleasure loop with the prefrontal cortex to keep you going on with the task.

But, beware of the dorsal striatum habit center telling you to keep procrastinating by watching video clips, texting, and checking emails. Counter this bad action with the prefrontal cortex, which is always trying to do the right thing, including meeting goals and avoiding procrastination. Keep the prefrontal cortex healthy and alert.

How do you keep the prefrontal cortex vigilant? Practice the attributes of well-being, such as always being engaged in life, finding meaning beyond yourself, and positive social interactions. Practice the ten health habits, such as eating healthy foods, sleeping for eight hours, exercising for one hour, learning something new every day, creating alpha-brainwave meditation time, and activating self-healing. Smile, it keeps the prefrontal cortex happy.

CHAPTER 16
BE YOUR TRUE SELF

Be yourself. It's freedom. It's freedom from reacting to criticism, freedom from blaming others, freedom from making excuses, and freedom from bad decisions. You don't have to react to criticism because your actions are your own, this is your character, and this is who you are.

You don't need to blame anyone else for what happens to you. All of your actions, good or bad, are your own. No need to blame an outside source. You don't need to make excuses. You don't make bad decisions, they're yours. Sometimes, the outcomes may be bad, but you can fix them.

Learn how to be your true self and experience total freedom. For me, I discovered a parasite while in medical school, a lung disease soon after, and I discovered how to improve people's lives all over the world. Along the way, I discovered myself, which was the best discovery of all.

You do not want to be who your parents wanted you to be, who your teachers and professors want you to be, who your boss wants you to be, or who society wants you to be. You do not want to be that unattainable person you've created in your mind that you will never be.

You want to discover and be the real you. Keep in mind that the person you discover is not static and fixed but alive in a state of flux with invigorating change. Be yourself. This gives you freedom from unnecessary decisions and stress, and the freedom to live life the way you want.

Finding your way to being your true self is a complex goal with no set timeline. For some people it happens in their 30s or 40s and for others in their 50s or 60s, and for some, never. It won't happen to anyone during their teenage years or during their early 20s because the prefrontal cortex required has not been fully developed. There is no easy five-step process for finding yourself because everyone is unique.

Maximize the components of well-being as a beginning for finding your true self. Set up your life in such a way that you will experience happy feelings, be engaged in life, create meaning in your life, and experience daily accomplishments.

Practicing the health habits will support your ability to become your true self, including the love of life, healthy nutrition, eight hours of sleep, one hour of continuous exercise, learning something new every day, alpha-brainwave meditation time every day, compassion, gratitude, and self-healing.

A major component of the journey of discovery is forgetting about your past failures and developing neuropathways to eliminate them from your conscious thinking. The only thing that makes them failures is your mind – comparing yourself to others, listening to people telling you that your actions are failures, and believing society, which has deemed your actions as failures.

They're not failures. They are something that you did or that happened to you that had a bad outcome. It's a bad outcome that needs to be forgotten.

Don't think about them. Don't allow the second thought. Don't allow the third thought reviewing the agonizing story cementing a negative neuropathway.

The negative energy is taking you away from making decisions. Or worse, you become afraid to make a decision or do anything because you don't want to repeat having the feeling of failure. This is in your mind – and the worst failure for one person may be an everyday minor failure for someone else.

Use the neurolinguistic bypass technique for these situations. Think about the event, develop the feeling of anguish in your stomach, say "love and peace" over and over for two minutes every morning for two weeks. After several days, you will not be able to create the painful feeling in your stomach when thinking about the event, and eventually the event and bitter feeling will be eliminated from your conscious mind, and allow you to learn to be yourself.

Do not accept what other people, books, blogs, or society consider to be your faults or weaknesses. Your traits are you. Embrace them and accept them.

You're too slow, you're too fast, you're late, you make mistakes, you're too quiet, you're too loud, you're too pushy, you're too passive, you're too mean, or you're too nice. These are your traits, whatever they are. This is who you are. Accept all of your behavior. Set your life up so you can use your traits. If you want to change one of them, go ahead, but do it because you want to change, not because of an outside force. This will help you be your true self and allow you to go forward with the life you want.

Associate yourself with upbeat, positive, and optimistic people who will not drain your energy. Listening to someone complain, make excuses, blame others, and criticize is a bad and depressing experience. You don't need this during your day. It not only uses up your energy, it leaves you depressed and without motivation. Associating with positive people makes it easier to be yourself in any situation.

Consider the subconscious mind when being your true self. Our physical actions are on automatic pilot at the subconscious level, which is a good thing so we don't have to decide to move the right foot forward and then the left foot forward while walking.

Although it feels like we make decisions about our behavior at the conscious level, we actually make them at the subconscious level. And if you are not aligned with your subconscious mind, unwanted behavior becomes a problem.

For example, driving doesn't require conscious decisions. It's all done by your subconscious mind without conscious thought. Here's a different type of example: you make an afternoon decision that you won't have dessert later on at the restaurant. You finish dinner and are asked whether you want to see the dessert menu. You say to yourself, *no I'm not going to have dessert,* but you instantly say, "Sure, I'll take a look." And, of course, you find something you want to order, and then you complain to yourself and feel guilty the whole time you're eating the dessert. This is not healthy. Combining a sugary dessert with stress produces a bad outcome.

You need to know that your subconscious mind is in charge of making all behavioral decisions. You decided not to have a dessert at the conscious level, but not at the subconscious level where a conditioned decision was made that had been established for years, probably during childhood. The subconscious mind always wins.

We now have the science to prove this. If you can understand this information and apply the understanding, it can have a profound positive effect on your behaviors and your life.

Professor Peter M. Vishton at William & Mary tells the clock-face story in his "Outsmart Yourself" lecture series. A study of people looking at a clock face and asked to randomly lift their right hand showed that a decision to move their right hand is made in the brain subconscious 300 milliseconds before the conscious decision is made.

People presume they make a conscious decision to move their right hand, and the brain instructs the muscles to carry it out. This experiment shows this presumption is wrong. The accurate sequence is the *subconscious* mind makes the decision and sends the signal to the motor system to carry out the action and sends a signal to the conscious mind to make it aware of the decision.

Another study confirmed that the subconscious mind controls decision making. People were asked to look at a photograph of a person and decide if the person looked pleasant or sinister. If they thought the person had a pleasant look, they pressed a right-hand clicker, and if they thought the person had a sinister look, they pressed a left-hand clicker.

The results of this study showed the decision is made at the subconscious level first, and not by milliseconds, but by seconds – so much time that the observer could tell which button was going to be pushed seconds before the person was aware of the action.

Furthermore, when the experimenters tricked the brain by changing the signal at the subconscious level, which made the person press the other button, the person showed no emotional response. This should have caused a panic reaction. When asked what happened, people responded casually by saying they changed their mind. People didn't change their mind, the experimenter did, which once again confirmed that the sub-conscious mind makes the decision and sends a message to the conscious mind signaling what decision was made.

How do these findings help you learn about being your true self? They make it clear that you must be in alignment with your subconscious mind to make healthy behavior decisions. Behavior decisions include choices you make about your health, career, and marriage. These are life-altering decisions, and making the right decisions leads to a healthy and enjoyable life.

Now that you know you must be aligned with the subconscious mind because it's in charge, how do you do this?

It's very difficult. We don't know what the subconscious mind is doing because it's not available to our conscious thinking. If your con-scious mind says no and your subconscious says yes to a behavior deci-sion, there's going to be frustration, anger, guilt, and more harm than good. Learn to be in alignment.

The reason the subconscious mind is not available to you is that more than 99 percent of the time, you are making desirable automatic deci-sions like walking, talking, driving, and eating. It's the one percent of decisions about behavior that we need to know about.

How do we communicate with the subconscious mind? It would be easy if we could use our words, but as you now know, it doesn't work that way. Your subconscious mind is telling you what to think, not the other way around. It's a one-way street.

You need to develop ways to communicate with the subconscious mind without words. One way to align yourself with the subconscious mind is during alpha- and theta-brainwave meditation. The conscious mind and subconscious mind merge together.

The subconscious mind is primitive. Like a crocodile brain, it responds to positive and negative reinforcement techniques. Therefore, use positive behavioral conditioning by stimulating dopamine release to the nucleus accumbens pleasure center of the brain through images, sounds, taste, smell, and touch.

For example, you have a bad habit of chewing gum in a social setting, biting your fingernails, or other unwanted minor habit. Your conscious mind knows this and wants to stop, but your subconscious mind tells you to continue because it gives you pleasure. It sends a surge of dopamine to the nucleus accumbens.

One way to change this behavior is to substitute a healthy alternative that will produce the dopamine response for the accumbens pleasure center. Reward yourself with something that gives you pleasure, such as a positive thought like love and peace. This reward is not for the conscious mind. It's for the subconscious mind.

If a reward is given for not doing a bad habit, the subconscious mind will not do the bad habit. This reward system is subtle and takes a long time to instill, but it can produce a permanent change for the better.

To show that the subconscious mind thinks automatically without conscious awareness, consider the subconscious mind as a "houseguest" who is a wonderful addition, bringing joy to your life and making your life better 99 percent of the time. But the remaining one percent of the time, your subconscious mind is an unruly guest, staying up late, making a mess out of the house, eating too much, eating bad foods, and disrupting your life with other bad habits. This guest is not going to change any of these behaviors, so you need to find a way to change them.

This is where communicating directly to the subconscious with images can be effective.

Use food as an example of effective imagery communication with the subconscious. People eat less food if the kitchen is clean. A dirty, untidy kitchen causes stress, and people eat more when stressed. Eat in a clean kitchen. People will eat less and digestion will be more efficient for a healthy life.

Use opaque containers for unhealthy foods and people will eat less of these foods because they cannot easily visualize them. Out of sight, out of mind.

Use small plates and bowls. The subconscious mind has established a set amount of food that should be on a plate, so using smaller plates results in a smaller amount of food that will be eaten with no change in the feeling of satisfaction. Use tall, thin glasses for beverages; less of the beverage will be consumed than if short, wide glasses are used.

Visualization is a way to communicate with the subconscious mind. There is no language involved, and there is a direct primitive brain connection with visualization.

Visualize the process, not the goal. You know the goal so no need to think about it or to spend time visualizing the outcome. Thinking about the goal is stressful and not attaining the goal day after day is not good, a bad feeling in the stomach.

Thinking about the process is a continuous feeling of accomplishment and engagement not associated with failure or success. It's not a competition with yourself to reach a goal. Thinking about the process produces a comforting sense of well-being.

Become your true self. It's the ultimate freedom. It gives you full confidence in yourself. Comparison with other people is destructive and takes away from who you are. You will be free from criticism, blame, and harsh words because your actions are your own and no excuses are needed. Make a mistake? Fix it. Don't beat yourself up.

Be yourself for the best feeling in the world.

CHAPTER 17
OPTIMISM

Optimism feels good. For centuries visitors have observed the boundless optimism among the people of the United States from one end of the country to the other. During the early 1800s, the visiting French author Alexis de Tocqueville wrote that optimism is a true American characteristic. In 2001, the Irish philosopher Charles Handy retraced Tocqueville's trek across America and was struck by the "energy, enthusiasm, and confidence in the country." He wrote that Americans "believe the future will be better," and they'll do whatever it takes to make it that way.

One Japanese guide for American culture noted that "In America, you can make mistakes, fail, and it doesn't matter. It's a fundamental feeling that to sometimes be incorrect is natural ... rather than thinking about mistakes and failures, Americans have curiosity and say, 'Let's try anyway!'"

Martin Seligman wrote the book *Learned Optimism* and found that optimists achieve more and have better overall health, while pessimists are prone to give up easier and are more prone to depression.

How to learn to be an optimist? Look at things in the right way. Obstacles and problems are brief setbacks, not permanent deterrents. Make positive generalizations. Something happens, it's not personal.

Events are temporary, not permanent. Optimistic people believe bad events are temporary and not permanent; therefore, they bounce back quickly from failure, while pessimists take longer periods to recover or, worse, may never recover.

Optimists think of positive, good events as permanent, while pessimists think of good things as transient. In contrast, optimists think of negative, bad events as transient and pessimists think of negative events as permanent.

Make positive generalizations. Optimists generalize good events to all parts of their lives while pessimists generalize an isolated failure in their lives as total failure.

Events are not personal. Optimists look for causes outside of themselves while pessimists take things personally, thinking they are the cause of a negative event.

Pessimists can learn a new way to respond to events. Good events are permanent. Bad events are transient and not permanent. An isolated failure is not a total failure. Events are not personal. Stop the second negative thought that leads to the third repeating the long, depressing story. Maximize the 15 lifestyle elements for optimistic thinking leading to an enjoyable and successful life.

CHAPTER 18
YOU'RE THE BOSS:
MANAGE YOUR DISEASE

Have you been diagnosed with a disease? Had an injury? Remember, you are in charge. You can manage your disease better than anyone else can. Learn the five steps to managing your disease or injury based on ideas that are familiar to you:

- First, learn everything you can about the disease or injury.
- Second, understand the risks and benefits of diagnostic procedures.
- Third, know the risks and benefits of treatment options.
- Fourth, establish a monitoring system.
- Fifth, create an environment for healing.

Let's start by understanding your relationship with disease. People often think of disease as an evil that must be eliminated. This is a successful strategy for some acute illnesses – treat the pneumonia with a powerful antibiotic that results in a cure. The problem is identified and stopped by the properly chosen solution. In these situations, the disease is a temporary annoyance in an otherwise normal life, readily replaced by the week's sporting event, a day at the beach, or an exhilarating experience at work, and then completely forgotten.

For chronic diseases, search and destroy tactics may do more harm than good. They may delay resolution of symptoms, and all too often lead to death.

———

Meet Joe and find out what happens when someone decides to search for total elimination. One morning as he was getting ready for work, Joe bent over to retrieve his shoes from under the bed. Almost immediately, he felt an excruciating pain in his lower back that radiated to his entire body. He crawled to a chair, angry and frustrated by the disabling pain.

Most of us have experienced something similar at one time or another during our lives. It's what we do next that will determine the difference between resolution and a life filled with misery.

Joe did what many people do. He couldn't go to work so he went to the emergency room.

"We have a low-back pain," the triage nurse told the ER doc in a flat tone of voice.

"Get some X-rays, and I'll see him," the doc said casually.

After looking at the CT scan, the doctor told Joe, "There seems to be something in the lower back."

These are ordinary words on the surface, but what does "something" mean? It usually means that the doctor sees a shadow or density that is a little out of the normal range, but nothing definite that can be labeled as an abnormality. The configuration of the lower back is such that almost everyone has a little "something" between or around the vertebral discs, findings that show no direct correlation with low-back pain.

"What do I do, Doctor?" Joe asked, grimacing in pain.

"Take these pain-relief tablets, anti-inflammatory pills, and stay flat on your back for six weeks," the doctor said confidently.

Joe did what he was told. He lay in bed with a board under the mattress for several days, and the pain disappeared. He continued for the prescribed six weeks, then suddenly developed pain in the right side of his chest. He didn't think it was a heart attack, but he called 911 for an ambulance because he could hardly talk due to shortness of breath.

This time, the ER acute-trauma team met Joe at the hospital entrance and rushed him to the ICU, where it was determined that his inactivity had resulted in pooling of the blood in his legs. The pooled blood formed blood clots that traveled to his lungs. He was given intravenous heparin.

After recovering, Joe did well for several months, then the back pain returned. He bypassed the ER this time and went directly to the orthopedic surgeon.

"We can fix this using our new mini-operation," the surgeon said enthusiastically. We'll use small two-inch tape to cover the incision. You'll be up and around the next day."

Joe liked this idea. In his mind, he heard this was fast, easy, and guaranteed to fix the low-back pain; all words of caution were not heard. He completed a mountain of paperwork and underwent the preoperative evaluation. He checked into the hospital at 5:30 the next morning. The nurses prepped him for surgery, and the anesthesiologist deftly inserted an intravenous line. The surgical checklist was completed in the operating room. The operation went smoothly, without a hint of a problem.

For the first time in weeks, Joe awoke with no pain. He had a smile that wouldn't quit. "This is fantastic!" he exclaimed, relieved and excited. He gradually returned to his normal activities, and memory of the low-back-pain agony faded.

But the story isn't over. Within a few months, Joe noticed an intermittent, annoying, dull ache in his lower back. The pain would come and go without interfering too much with his daily activities. But, he soon convinced himself that even this occasional pain had to be stopped.

So obsessed did he become with eliminating the pain that he soon became filled with anger and rage. He talked to anyone who would listen. "It's an excruciating, throbbing, knife-in-the-back pain. You have no idea what it's like to have this crushing pain day after day after day," Joe moaned.

He wasn't aware that each time he used these words and told his anguished story, he was establishing a new neurolinguistic pain pathway. Neurolinguistics refers to the connection between words and the brain. If you continually say negative words, you will eventually establish harmful thinking pathways that, over time, change who you are and how you act. This can also occur in relation to pain. If you use words such as *agonizing, unbearable,* and *crushing* to describe your pain, over and over, you will eventually establish a pathway so ingrained in your brain that the pain becomes real.

Studies have now shown that your word choice can cause disease. Marty Seligman's team explored people's "word cloud", the words people use in their social media sites, and found that the word cloud is a better predictor of heart disease than traditional risk factors such as smoking, diabetes, and hypertension. Thinking, talking and using negative words every day and night can be harmful and even deadly.

It's important to build a positive neurolinguistic pathway by uses beneficial phrases, such as "the pain is manageable" and "the pain can be controlled."

If the negative neurolinguistic pathway has been established, build a neuropathway bypass to override the dysfunctional pathway by not using negative words and replacing them with positive words and phrases.

Joe didn't know that he was perpetuating the pain in a vicious feedback loop that zapped any hope of resolution. He didn't know about neurolinguistics, and he didn't care. He had to eliminate the pain at all costs.

Joe had heard about acupuncture, and it sounded good. He endured multiple visits and insertions of needles throughout his body. He was pleasantly surprised to find relief from the pain.

Yet several weeks after his final visit, the mild intermittent lower-back pain returned.

Joe once again convinced himself the pain was excruciating and freely told everyone the agonies of his life. His wife was becoming more and more annoyed with his incessant grumbling. His friends had had enough of it as well and avoided him. Joe solved the problem by finding new friends who complained about their problems as much as he did. This only perpetuated his pain.

Joe was now more determined than ever to annihilate the pain. His wish apparently came true when he visited a pain-management anesthesiologist, who told him that a nerve block would stop the pain. Joe signed the consent form without a thought, again ignoring all words of caution, and the procedure was performed.

The pain was gone once again. Soon, Joe realized that somewhere along the way he had acquired a morphine pump that he could use at any time, and he did so freely at the smallest hint of pain.

Months passed. Joe had become depressed and addicted to morphine. He lost his wife, his job, and his income. He was more obsessed than ever about stopping the pain, even if it registered only one on a scale of one to ten.

What do you think happened to Joe? There are several possible outcomes, including death due to a catastrophic medical procedure or a drug-resistant infection or suicide.

Do you know someone like him? What happened to Joe is happening to people around the world every day – not only those with low-back pain but with hundreds of other ailments.

There is another way. By taking charge, Joe could have had a successful outcome without intense medications, surgery, drug addiction, and loss of his job and family.

Mary managed her low-back pain the right way. One day while working out at her gym, she awkwardly reached down to retrieve a set of light dumbbells and twisted her lower back. The sudden and excruciating pain radiated all the way down to her right toe. It hurt so much that she almost fainted. But Mary realized that the pain was part of her and not something to fight. So she sought out the gym's trainer, who provided deep-muscle back therapy for athletes.

After a muscle treatment, Mary's pain improved somewhat, and she was able to do what she needed to do throughout the day, albeit slowly and cautiously. That night, however, was a different story. Once in bed, Mary struggled to find a comfortable position. Somehow she managed to get enough sleep.

The next day, as the injured cells in the lower back had created more inflammation, she was in even more pain. She read everything she could about low-back pain. She found out about the types of diagnostic studies and when they were needed. And she learned that the second day may be worse because toxic substances released by the inflamed cells may cause increased pain. Therefore, she continued her plan of cautious ambulation, and she was able to accomplish most of the things that needed her attention.

Another low-back muscle treatment seemed to improve the situation, as the spasmodic muscles had lessened their grip on the nerves exiting her lower spine. The pain and numbness in her right toe had decreased. She slept better that night.

The next day, she was able to increase her activities. Within several days, she was almost back to normal. She felt so much better that she returned to the gym. Exercising at a slow and deliberate pace, she was able to complete her workout routine.

After three months, she was pain-free and actively living her life again. She began incorporating exercises to strengthen her core abdominal and back muscles into her workout. The pain occurred again several months later, but thanks to hip flexor stretching and core muscle exercises, the pain was relieved within 48 hours. Mary continued her core-strengthening exercises, and the disabling pain did not recur.

The important lesson is that you and the disease or injury are connected. The disease is part of you. It's not a healthy or pleasant part, and it wreaks havoc on your life, but it's part of you.

Sometimes disease is caused by an external force, such as a microorganism that has invaded the system, and antibiotics will cure the problem. Sometimes it's a growth than can be cut out and discarded. Often, however, it's chronic and without known cause.

Mary followed the five steps of managing her low-back pain. Joe did not.

Joe failed to learn anything about low-back pain; Mary learned as much as she could. Joe didn't ask about diagnostic tests or what they would show; Mary studied the causes of low-back pain and learned about the diagnostic process. Joe concentrated on the benefits of the treatment options and paid no attention to the risks. He didn't find out about the natural course of typical low-back pain. Mary studied the treatment management options and realized that the tensed, spasmodic muscles were pulling the nerves, thereby aggravating the pain. She knew that low-back pain eventually subsides in the vast majority of people.

Joe had no monitoring system; Mary monitored her symptoms, knowing the expected course of the discomfort.

Joe failed in every way possible to create an environment in which he could heal. He approached the pain as an evil force that had to be stopped. He continually complained. He sought any treatment he could find to stop the pain. He developed no preventive management.

Mary did the opposite. She approached the situation in a positive manner. She considered it manageable and did not allow it to consume her life. She developed a program to strengthen her back muscles and prevent future episodes.

Many types of heart, lung, kidney, liver, skeletal muscular, and neurological diseases are chronic, as are some cancers, and most do not have an established cause. They may not be curable, but you can take charge and learn to manage them, allowing you to live an active, enjoyable life.

The first step in managing your disease is to learn everything you can about the disease process. Learn everything about what you're facing. Learn what it is, what caused it, diagnostic and treatment options, and importantly, its natural course. What happens if pills, surgery, or other medical interventions are not used?

Ask your doctor, but don't stop there. Read about it and do research. Explore academic university-based internet sites to discover facts about the disease process or injury. Ask questions in discussion forums. You will find people all over the world with similar issues. You'll be able to talk to people who have very rare diseases. You'll find out how they learn to manage their disease.

———

Let's follow Dr. Roberts through the five steps of managing his disease.

It had been a typical day, filled with work and enjoyable family activities, for Dr. Roberts, a prominent Massachusetts physician. Now he was looking forward to a relaxing evening with his family. Sadly, that wasn't to be.

Suddenly, as he was finishing dinner with his wife, Susanne, and his two sons, Colby and Brent, he felt a sharp, stabbing pain in the pit of his stomach. He finished the last bite of dessert, hoping to relieve the pain. Bad idea, it didn't work.

"It's indigestion," he grumbled to himself." He ignored the pain and helped the kids with their homework. The pain worsened relentlessly, traveling straight to his back. Sips of water and doses of antacids had no effect. Finally, at midnight, he threw up.

Mercifully, the pain stopped. Dr. Roberts dragged himself to bed and drifted off into a deep but short-lived sleep. Two hours later he awoke, doubled over with pain. Soon he was writhing on the bathroom floor, hugging the toilet bowl.

He woke up his wife and told her he was going to the 24-hour drugstore for something stronger than an antacid. By the time he returned home, the pain was unbearable, ten on a one-to-ten-point scale. By 6 a.m., chills had started. For the first time in his married life, he asked Susanne, "Could you get me to the hospital?"

He threw up one more time, which gave him some relief. They then packed the kids into the car and dropped them off at school.

Dr. Roberts endured the 40-minute drive to the hospital where he had his practice. By the time they arrived, he was in agony. He was bent over in pain as he walked down the hall to the observation unit, where he was put on a stretcher. Intravenous fluids were started.

It was nice to see a friendly face as the gastroenterologist, a coworker, arrived. Then the surgeon, his good friend and colleague, showed up. Dr. Roberts thought his friend had just stopped by to say hello.

"It's gastritis," Dr. Roberts kept thinking to himself. Then, before he knew what was happening, the skilled hands of the surgeon began to examine his belly.

The doctors left the room. When they returned, the surgeon said, "You probably have a perforated ulcer." Dr. Roberts was in complete disbelief. An ulcer? He had never had an ulcer. He had never even had symptoms associated with an ulcer. He had always been in good health. Maybe the doctors were right. In medical school he had learned that a rigid abdomen and excruciating pain that went straight to the back were symptoms of an ulcer.

As Dr. Roberts sat in a wheelchair, waiting to be taken for an X-ray, he had reached a desperate state. His abdomen was in a violent uproar. He was severely nauseated. He had chills. He thought he had developed an infection and was going into shock.

Turning to his wife, he said, "I feel like I'm dying." Dramatically, he added, "If anything happens to me, promise you won't let them put me on a breathing machine."

Dr. Roberts was in the first step of managing his disease: he was trying to learn as much as possible about it. In an acute, life-threatening situation, the first thing to do is to ask the doctor for information. In a chronic, ongoing situation, first ask the doctor, then search the internet, read a book or an e-book, listen to a CD, or participate in an interactive program.

Learn everything that you can, and keep on learning. The information will help you to control the situation and to make the decisions that are best for you.

The second step in managing your disease is to understand the risks and benefits of diagnostic procedures. You will be asked an organized series of questions designed to lead to the diagnosis. You will have a physical examination searching for clues. After this, you will have a sequential group of diagnostic tests and procedures.

Let's start with the questions you'll be asked. In many situations, the diagnosis can be revealed by asking questions, and it can be confirmed during an examination and other diagnostic procedures.

The questions begin with your chief complaint, what brought to the office today? The remaining questions are designed to arrive at the most likely possibility. You'll be asked about diseases that might have occurred in your family, such as heart disease, high blood pressure, diabetes, asthma, allergies, or cancer. Some diseases run in families, so this information helps to confirm a diagnostic possibility. You'll also be asked about your own medical conditions. Questions about your home life will be posed as well.

You'll be asked if you drink alcohol, and if so, what types, how much, and how frequently. Sometimes the four CAGE questions will be asked. *C* is for cut down. Have you ever felt you should cut down on your drinking? *A* is for annoyed. Have people annoyed you by criticizing your drinking? *G* is for guilty. Have you ever felt bad or guilty about your drinking? *E* is for eye-opener. Have you ever had a drink first thing in the morning to steady your nerves or get rid of a hangover? The answers to these questions can be used to determine whether an individual is alcohol-dependent, and the symptoms or findings may be related to underlying complications of alcoholism.

Questions about occupational and environmental exposure will come next. You will routinely be asked about allergies and adverse drug reactions. The final part of the questions component focuses on medications that you might be taking. It's helpful to know the name of each medication, the dose, when it was started, and the reason for taking it, because medications can have unusual side effects that could be the cause of the current problem.

———

Harold was taking warfarin, a blood-thinning medication designed to prevent blood clots, because of his irregular heart rate. "I've developed a nasty cough, and I'm bringing up green phlegm," he told the doctor who was on call during the weekend. His symptoms had become worrisome.

"I'll meet you at the ambulatory care center," the doctor replied.

"Sounds like you have bronchitis," the doctor said, after listening to Harold's lungs. "Let's put you on a five-day course of azithromycin."

Three days later, the cough and phlegm were gone, but Harold had other problems. So he called his regular physician, Dr. Burns. "I'm having a nosebleed, and I have bruises on my hands," he told the doctor, somewhat alarmed.

"I'm pleased to hear about the resolution of your bronchitis, but I'm concerned about your nosebleed. Come in for a blood test to find out about your warfarin level," Dr. Burns told him.

"Oops, I forgot to tell the doctor over the weekend about taking warfarin," Harold sheepishly told Dr. Burns.

"Azithromycin is metabolized by a specialized liver enzyme and is one of the medications that can increase the effectiveness of warfarin. So your blood is much thinner than we like to have it," Dr. Burns explained.

The laboratory test confirmed that Harold's blood was too thin, but by taking less warfarin for a few days, serious complications were averted.

The physical examination comes next. Your vital signs will be taken. Your heart and lungs will be examined for abnormalities. Specific heart sounds, like a third (extra) heart sound from congestive heart failure or the swooshing sound of abnormal heart valves, could be the result of underlying disease. Certain lung sounds, like wheezing, may indicate asthma, while crackles may be due to pneumonia. Next, your abdomen will be examined for abnormal masses and to determine whether your liver or spleen is enlarged. The extent of the physical examination is directed by the symptoms. An intense and detailed examination of the system associated with the symptoms will be conducted.

Sarah felt a lump on the left side of her abdomen just below her ribs, but she wasn't sick and didn't have symptoms.

Dr. Strong examined her eyes, ears, nose, and throat and found them to be normal; however, several lymph nodes in her neck were enlarged. Her lungs had normal breath sounds, and there were no wheezes or crackles. The heart examination found a regular heart rate without murmurs. The neurological examination was normal.

Dr. Strong examined Sarah's abdomen and confirmed her impression of an abnormality, an enlarged spleen.

"Why is my spleen enlarged?" Sarah asked.

"It's an unusual finding by itself," Dr. Strong replied. "In many parts of the world, it's common and indicates malarial infection."

Sarah was puzzled as to how she could have contracted malaria. "I haven't traveled outside of my home in Minnesota for several months, and I haven't visited any countries where malaria occurs."

"An enlarged spleen could be caused by lymphoma, but there are usually other symptoms," Dr. Strong said.

"But I've felt great," Sarah answered energetically. "I haven't had a fever, night sweats, loss of appetite, or weight loss."

"Remember I told you that I felt some enlarged lymph nodes in your neck?" the doctor asked.

"Yes, what does that mean?"

"Combined with the enlarged spleen, they most likely show that you have sarcoidosis," Dr. Strong answered.

Sarcoidosis is a chronic disorder of unknown cause in which immune-system cells cluster to form small swirls of tissue called *granulomas*. These formations usually occur in the lungs, but they may develop in any organ system in the body, including lymph nodes, spleen, liver, and skin. Ultimately, Dr. Strong confirmed this diagnosis. In most people, the disease will disappear without treatment, but others need corticosteroid medication.

Dr. Strong and Sarah monitored the symptoms, and over the next year the disease resolved without treatment.

———

After taking a history and performing a physical examination, diagnostic tests will be done. You may consider this a perfunctory step, yet, it's important that you pay attention and learn everything you can about this part of the diagnostic process.

Ask questions. Are tests necessary, and if so, why? Is it necessary to obtain a CT or MRI scan? If so, what are the expected results? Is there a wide range of normal findings? Do the findings correlate with the disease process? Will dye be used? Are you allergic to the dye?

What are the benefits of the diagnostic test? Are there false-positive tests – tests that show positive findings even though there's nothing abnormal? Conversely, what is the chance that the test will not establish the diagnosis? Is it worth performing the test? Answers to these questions will provide information that will help you to make the best decision.

Similar questions can be asked about blood tests. Even though blood tests are routine and cause only fleeting discomfort, some are expensive and the diagnostic yield so small that they should not be performed.

In addition, nonspecific tests may show an unexpected abnormal result that will prompt further testing. In some situations, a biopsy will be performed, with potential complications leading to a disastrous result, a price too high for a random abnormality with no specific symptoms.

For example, typical laboratory tests are based on finding the normal value in hundreds of thousands of healthy individuals. Abnormal tests are determined by the values outside the 95 percent range, which means that 5 percent of people have an abnormal test even though they are healthy. So if you have 20 tests, one may be considered abnormal but may actually represent a healthy individual. These findings cannot be ignored, as it is not known whether the test is abnormal because of disease or whether the person is part of the healthy population.

A repeat test and monitoring is often a good approach. If the value remains at the same level over time, this is within the healthy-population group and there is no need for additional, potentially dangerous diagnostic procedures. If the value increases or decreases, the test often reflects a specific underlying cause, which can be further evaluated.

Obtaining diagnostic tests for a specific diagnosis is needed. Nonspecific random testing that searches for a nonspecific diagnosis often leads to confusion, a poor diagnostic yield, and wasted time. Find out the specific reason for the test, and if it makes sense to you, proceed with it.

Tissue biopsies are a special consideration. Collection of biopsy tissue is the most definitive method of establishing a correct diagnosis, and it remains the best method available for diagnosing many diseases, such as cancer and obscure connective-tissue or immunological disorders.

Some of these procedures, such as a skin biopsy with use of local anesthesia, are minor and only slightly uncomfortable, although they will leave a small scar. Other minor biopsies include lymph-node procedures, which can be conducted near the surface of the skin with local anesthesia, leaving a longer scar. Some biopsies, such as liver and kidney biopsies, can be performed with a needle. Other biopsies, such as lung, heart, and brain biopsies, require major surgery. These procedures can be helpful in establishing a diagnosis so that the correct treatment can be given, especially in lymphoma or rare immunological conditions.

Some individuals who have had diagnostic biopsies never seem to recover. The tendency is to blame the procedure for the deterioration, but the association is usually coincidental: a person may have been ill with a disorder for a long time that did not respond to medical treatment. The biopsy did not affect the course of the illness.

Tissue biopsy is often an essential part of the diagnostic process. Ask the doctor or surgeon about the reason for the biopsy and the risks of the procedure.

———

My friend Jim asked me to look at a rash. That's a question you don't want to hear in the gym locker room, but I trusted Jim and took a look. It was a big red circle behind his knee.

"Could this be Lyme disease?" he asked. "I saw a tick on my dog a few days ago, but the doctor told me there was no white center in the rash, so it probably wasn't Lyme disease."

There were several options. This could be a topical allergic reaction treatable with a lotion. He could see a dermatologist. He could wait a couple of days to see if the rash went away. But, waiting could be a major problem. If this was Lyme disease, the rash would disappear in a few days, but the bacteria spirochete would continue to live, causing serious chronic heart and brain consequences.

The scenario should have played out like this: Jim has a diagnostic blood test that morning after leaving the gym. The test requires time and inconvenience, discomfort from a blood test, and an expense, but it could save his life. Lyme disease treated early is virtually always curable. Lyme disease treated late has deadly consequences. Jim sees me a few days later during my workout and tells me the test was positive, and he is completing his treatment. I am grateful to hear the news and grateful he was treated early.

However, in reality, Jim did not have a pleasing story to tell me. He was not able to be tested that morning nor the next day nor the next. He made multiple and repeated telephone calls, but no one would see him that day and he wasn't able to get an appointment for two weeks. He sent pictures, and was told no white center, so no test. When he was finally able to have the test, the doctor's face blanched after looking at the rounded red rash without the white center and the positive test result. Treatment was started immediately.

The lesson? During Lyme disease season, if you have a rash or unusual insect bite – or are worried that you may have been bitten by a tick and think there's *any possibility* that you have Lyme disease – **get a test**. It will be inconvenient, take time and probably some money, cause a little discomfort, and if negative, upset someone in the health-care system. But, a positive test will save your life.

––––––

Let's return to Dr. Roberts for the diagnostic process. An abdominal X-ray was the next obvious diagnostic step. It was ordered to help determine whether there was air in the abdomen, which would clinch the diagnosis of a ripped and gashed stomach from a perforated ulcer.

The abdominal X-ray showed no air under the diaphragm. This was good news, as it meant no leaky stomach from an ulcer and therefore no need for emergency surgery or intravenous antibiotics.

The analgesic began to take effect, and the pain began to subside. Maybe it had been indigestion after all.

In this setting, the pain was probably being numbed by the medication and would recur as the medication wore off.

So the next best step was to get an abdominal computerized tomography (CT) scan, which would provide a three-dimensional picture of the abdominal organs, revealing a tumor, gallbladder or kidney stones, or other diagnostic considerations. The risk of the CT scan is that it may show too much. Every tiny detail is seen with such precision that possible abnormalities are noted on almost everyone's scans. There is such a wide range of normal that many of these findings are neither indicative of disease nor abnormal.

However, in the acute situation of Dr. Roberts, the abdominal CT scan was the appropriate and best option, as there were major benefits with negligible risk. So he was wheeled to the CT suite for the scan.

After the study was completed, the chief of radiology came in with a look on his face that Dr. Roberts knew meant that something was terribly wrong.

"You have a bowel obstruction," the chief said reluctantly.

Dr. Roberts acknowledged this completely unexpected finding with a moment of silence. For the previous 16 hours, this relatively common diagnosis had never entered his mind. It should have, because he had anticipated this dreadful moment on countless occasions over the years – in medical school, while working in the jungles of the Amazon, and while taking care of patients in the plains of Africa – but it had not happened.

When Dr. Roberts was nine, like millions of other kids his age he had his appendix removed. Unknown to him, small rubber band–like scars called *adhesions* developed in his abdomen after the operation.

Three weeks after his appendectomy, he had a stomachache that wouldn't go away. Loops of the small bowel had gotten tangled in the adhesions and become obstructed. The blood supply was cut off and the bowel was dying. So he had another major operation that untangled the snarled bowel but left him weak and exhausted.

Three weeks after this surgery, the bowel once again became tangled, resulting in a third surgery. Shortly after recovering from this surgery, while he was eating a peanut-butter-and-jelly sandwich, his stomach began to hurt. He was sitting on the couch, looking out the window and waiting for his father to return from work. When his father walked through the door, he had a look of deep sadness and disappointment, knowing the reality that his son was again going to have to face surgery in what was now a desperately weakened condition. The bowel was again entangled, caught in the web of the freshly formed adhesions. This was the fourth major operation in just a few weeks' time.

Dr. Roberts remembered being sad and frightened by the many hospital ordeals, especially the part when the tube was inserted in his nose and down into his stomach, although he never considered the danger. Much later, he realized that, during the first few hours and days after that last surgery, his mother didn't think he would survive. It was so much in so little time for a young boy to go through. But he did get better; the bowel recovered. He went on to experience an invigorating and marvelous life, until this latest diagnosis.

Dr. Roberts had completed the second step in managing his disease. The diagnostic process had been accomplished successfully without harm. Now he needed to go to the next step.

The third step in managing your disease is to know the risk and benefits of the treatment options. There are always options. You now must begin the process of learning and understanding everything you can about your treatment options.

Every situation is unique, and one of the options is going to be best for you. The best evidence-based treatment option may be perfect for most people but may not be the best one for you.

Treatment options will depend on what type of health-care provider you're seeing. If you're seeing an internist, medicines will be discussed. If it's a surgeon, surgery will be the focus. If it's an herbalist, herbs will be the topic, while an acupuncturist will advocate acupuncture. Ask questions about the effectiveness and risks of the various treatments. Some people like to ask about the statistics of success. What are the alternatives? What are the benefits and side effects of the alternative treatments?

Important in these discussions is the natural history of the disease. What happens if you decide not to have treatment at this time? The answer will allow you to be in control of the situation and to make the decision that is best for you. For example, why would anyone refuse a life-saving operation? Almost always, the answer would be straightforward – surgery is the best option – but for people in very unusual situations it may not be.

Learn and understand all of the available information about the benefits and risks of treatment so that you can make the decision that is best for you, which is not necessarily what is best for the doctor.

———

Dr. Roberts' thoughts were interrupted as he was wheeled from the CT suite to the radiology corridor.

"You have a tangled bowel and probably strangled blood vessels," the surgeon said candidly. "The bowel will die as the loss of blood supply intensifies."

The surgeon recommended an immediate operation, with an incision down the middle of the belly. Dr. Roberts thought to himself that there had to be an alternative. In the back of his mind, he knew that if he had this operation, new adhesions would develop, resulting in the need for another surgery and leading to a continuous round of adhesions and operations. This time he might die.

"Is there another option?" he asked cautiously.

By then, his friend the gastroenterologist had arrived in the corridor. "There is another option," he said prudently. "The white-blood-cell count is increased but not too high. The abdomen is rigid but not too rigid. There is no fever. So let's monitor the situation, one hour at a time."

"Will this save my life?" Dr. Roberts wondered to himself.

It was a bold decision. No one in the world would have faulted the surgeon; an operation was clearly indicated. Fortunately, the surgeon's vast experience and discerning wisdom allowed him to agree to observation, and he responded, "One hour at a time."

Dr. Roberts was returned to his hospital room. A few minutes later, another friend and colleague came to visit. Dr. Roberts anticipated a few pleasant remarks and best wishes for a speedy recovery. What he received instead may have saved his life.

Unexpectedly, his friend quietly said a few vital words: "First, breathe with your stomach; it has a positive, relaxing effect. Second, visualize the problem, visualize the tangled bowel and vessels, and untangle them. Then divorce yourself from the traumatic and frightening events that happened when you were nine. That was then and this is now."

He gently added, "Have compassion for your stomach and intestines. Do not give them worry. Give them compassion." The friend's remarks and perception were based on seasoned knowledge and wisdom, as he was also the hospital minister and psychologist.

There are always treatment options. Find out everything you can about them. One is going to be best for you.

The fourth step in managing your disease is to establish a monitoring system. Now that you're receiving treatment, a monitoring system can save your life.

A successful monitoring system can be based on a series of three questions. Ask yourself: Are you feeling better? Are you feeling worse? Are you feeling the same?

If you are feeling better, stay with the same management. If you feel the same, keep going and follow the 48-hour rule – check again in 48 hours. If you are worse, reread the information about the disease process and review the diagnostic process and the treatment options. The next step will be obvious – a call to your doctor, a visit to the emergency room, or in some situations, the 48-hour rule – reevaluate.

The monitoring system can be as simple as reviewing the situation in your mind every couple of days. With chronic conditions, however, positive and negative changes may occur over weeks or months, so writing down the symptoms in a notebook or on a computer can be useful.

Choose two or three symptoms, enter your results into the computer, and create a graphic image of the disease so that you will have a color-coded visualization of its clinical course. The image will easily show one of three outcomes: you're improving, you're the same, or you're worse.

With this information, you can choose the course of action that is best for you. In many situations, the monitoring system itself can result in improvement, as daily discomforts are ignored, which eliminates potentially harmful visits for diagnostic studies or new treatments.

———

For Dr. Roberts, one hour passed, then two and three. Fever did not develop. The pain was controlled with a tube in his stomach and an occasional analgesic injection, but there were no tinkling sounds in the bowel. The silent bowel was potentially an ominous sign, as it remained twisted and snarled like a pot of spaghetti.

The next morning, another scan was ordered. The radiology chief convinced Dr. Roberts that it was necessary. Then he was told about the five giant cups of liquid he had to drink before the scan. To him it seemed like five gallons. It was something he did not want to do because the pain had stopped and the fluid would start the obstruction process over again – or would it? Maybe it would gently open the obstruction.

"Let's get started," the nurse said sternly but with compassion. The first cup went down grudgingly. Dr. Roberts immediately became nauseated and started sweating. He felt like he was again going into shock, but the nasty liquid stayed put. One cup down, four to go. He had a few minutes of rest. Down went another cup, and another, and another. Finally all five cups had vanished. It sounds like a simple process, but in this situation it was a monumental task.

The scan was performed while Dr. Roberts lay quietly on the gurney. The technologist took picture after picture. Dr. Roberts asked casually, "Did anything go through?"

The answer was on her face. "No," she said reluctantly.

It was noon now. Dr. Roberts was returned to his hospital room. Susanne had left to pick up the kids from school. He was alone. After the X-ray results, it was becoming clear that the entanglement was permanent. Dr. Roberts began preparing himself mentally for the surgery.

The fifth and final step in managing your disease is to create an environment for healing. Your body has an almost unlimited ability to heal itself. You have to know how to let this happen, as the ability may be dormant or blunted by the intensity of our daily lives. There are several basic tenets to healing. Some are from the soft, gentle sciences.

First, use a positive approach to the illness. This will allow you to have more energy, be compliant with the medication regimen, and take charge. Approaching the disease in a positive manner will also help you to avoid the neurolinguistic trap. Remember, repeatedly thinking about and verbalizing negative feelings about the illness will establish a new neuropathway that can send you down the road of perpetual aggravation of your symptoms and could make the situation even worse.

Second, use visualization. For example, visualize blood vessels and airways opening or healthy, strong joints. Visualizing healthy cells can make you feel more in control. Every cell in the body is continually replaced, some every few minutes and others every few weeks or months. Visualize healthy, strong cells replacing the inflamed or dysfunctional cells. Begin with replacing a few cells, but think big and ultimately visualize replacing millions. You can use this visualization process three times each day or anytime you wish. You can monitor the process with your disease-monitoring system.

Third, have overpowering confidence in yourself, your health-care providers, your family, your friends, and everyone at work. This will enhance the healing energy system of the body.

Fourth, have compassion for the diseased organ system. It's functionally perfectly well. The disease is causing the dysfunction, and the diseased cells can be replaced with healthy cells or, in situations of scarring, the healthy cells can become dominant.

Fifth, be persistent, as these methods require repetition and time, sometimes weeks or months.

The traditional sciences give us several potent tools to create an environment in which to heal: a sleep-hygiene program, healthy eating, a routine exercise program, and alpha-brainwave meditation.

Sleep is a traditional tool used to create an environment in which to heal. After years of study and despite exceptions, eight hours of sleep appears to be a requirement for a healthy life for the majority of people. Eight hours are required to regenerate the energy chemical adenosine that is used up during the day hours, and the last two hours are needed to obtain the full requirement of REM (rapid-eye movement) sleep. A healthy sleep-hygiene program consists of not allowing yourself to fall asleep watching television before you go to bed, going to bed and awakening at regular times, and not eating or eating very little three hours before you go to sleep.

Eat healthy foods that will not harm you. These include foods with no added sugar, no added salt, and no processed omega-6 fats. Food needs to be prepared in the right way and to be eaten in the right amount, at the right time.

Exercise through a rehabilitation program with physical and muscle therapy is important. The program will teach you about the basic aspects of the disease and will help you to design a weekly exercise program that you can do in your home or at any workout facility. The rehabilitation professionals can create an exercise that is best for your condition, whether it's post-surgery, arthritis, a heart problem, an intestinal disorder, or a lung condition.

Alpha-brainwave meditation time creates an environment to heal by decreasing stress, rebalancing the discordant realms of the brain, and producing feel-good hormones and neurotransmitters.

———

While Dr. Roberts was studying the surgery consent form, he had a compelling thought: *Maybe I can create an environment for healing, and I can heal myself.*

As his abdominal pain reached a level approaching nine on a scale of one to ten, he requested another injection of painkiller. Then, one by one, he relaxed each muscle. He breathed slowly and deeply with his abdomen. He visualized the uncoiling of his snarled bowel. He gave his bowel compassion. Every fiber and muscle in his body was relaxed.

He woke up two hours later. Everything was moving briskly once again. Dr. Roberts was cured. Whether there was a cause and effect or whether it was a naturally occurring event did not matter. An abdominal CT scan that afternoon confirmed it.

Now it was time for recovery. The next morning, he walked into the hall with the intravenous pole by his side. He sat on the exercise bicycle, slowly turning the pedals for a refreshing stretch. Two or three hours later, he fell asleep in a chair in the solarium, holding his wife's hand.

When he was back in his room, the gastroenterologist examined him and said confidently, "Let's pull out the stomach tube." Out it came. What a relief.

Miraculously, Dr. Robert's appetite returned in full force. He dreamt about food. He had his first taste of chicken broth, and it was heavenly. The second taste was not quite as exhilarating. The third taste was boring. But he was alive and ready to get out of there. By 2 p.m., after signing the necessary forms, he was on his way home.

By the time he walked into his house, the pangs of hunger were worse than any other symptom had been, so he ate some vanilla pudding and went to bed. He fell asleep for a while but woke up in a sweat with a vicious pain shooting across his abdomen. He walked downstairs, sat on the porch steps, and waited for Susanne to return, just as he had waited for his father many years earlier.

But this time it would be different. When Susanne, the kids, an uncle, and a grandmother arrived, the pain had become entrenched with an excruciating fierceness that nearly panicked him. Dr. Roberts was beginning to falter. He feared another cycle of hospitalizations.

Fortunately, he remembered the concept of creating an environment for healing. It was going to be hard work, but he believed that he would succeed. He followed his family into the house and headed straight for the family room and his son's piano keyboard. He put on the earphones, adjusted them, and began to play. He played all the Disney tunes he could remember, songs from *Phantom of the Opera,* and Mozart. The music began to heal him. It was magical. It was soothing.

He turned up the volume to drown out the tension that families sometimes create inadvertently. It worked. He played for an hour. Finally, the last of the pain was gone. Dr. Roberts had returned to normal.

The next morning, he awoke to a glorious early spring day. He went outside and sat on the porch, watching a blue jay share birdseed with a chipmunk. The chipmunk's cheeks were filled with seed. Other birds, including two red house wrens, also shared the seeds. This scene also became part of his healing.

Several years passed. Dr. Roberts' illness never came back. He continued his morning runs and began working out in the gym every day. He was stronger and healthier than when he was in medical school. He stopped eating fried food and kept food containing saturated fat to a minimum. He doubled the amount of soluble and insoluble fiber in his diet. At first, the fiber diet caused him some discomfort, but once his system became used to it, he experienced a feeling of improved health, vigor, and energy. His cholesterol was normal, and his weight was normal. Dr. Roberts was a happy, contented guy.

As it turned out, the disease was not the enemy. Dr. Roberts realized he could not fight it because it was a battle he could not win. So he managed it.

Remember, you can manage your disease better than anyone else can. Your chances of success are unlimited.

CHAPTER 19
LIVE TO 140

Why 140 years? During one of my morning workouts, my friend Scott asked me how long humans can live.

"140 years," I said instantly.

"Why 140?" he asked.

"Because it feels right, and it can be done now," I replied.

So began my journey to confirm this prediction. You will be surprised about what I found, and *Time* magazine agrees with me – the February 23, 2015 cover featured a picture of a baby that could live to be 142 years old.

The first question to ask: Do people want to live to 140?

The answer should be an obvious yes, but, surprisingly, the majority of people would say no. They cringe at the thought because since childhood, people have been conditioned through the subconscious mind to think that people in their 70s and 80s are old. Worse yet, in their minds, people over 100 are broken down, bent over, wrinkled, and shriveled up – and look like walking corpses. This is a powerful negative image. The image is so strong that people grow old and age this way because of their negative subconscious drives.

If people equate decline and decay with someone who is 90 or 100, they can't imagine how bad a 140-year-old person would look.

We have been conditioned to think of old-age people as being cranky, complaining, blaming others, and criticizing. When people get old, the future is painful and filled with problems. Old people develop age spots and wrinkles. Old people are supposed to retire and drop out of life.

These assumptions have been planted in our minds since childhood. But, none of them are true.

We have been conditioned to grow old and die. Within the next 24 hours, you're going to hear someone say one or more of the following: "I'm too old to do that." "I never want to grow old." "I dread my birthday, I'm a year older." "Wait until you're 50, your body is going to fall apart." You've heard the same thing said about turning 60 or 70, and even 30 or 40 from some people. No wonder people grow old and die, they're supposed to.

Think about living to 140 filled with vigor and energy. You're 40 years old, you have 100 years to live. If you're 70 years old, you've only lived one-half of your life! You have many, many years to live a life filled with joy, happiness, excitement, helping people, learning, creativity, and stimulating, invigorating experiences.

This is an astounding and exhilarating feeling. Look what you've accomplished so far. Look at the experiences you've had, the people you've met, the places you've been, and the discoveries you've made. You will meet new people who will enrich your life, see new places, experience new adventures, learn new ways of doing things, share your creativity, and much more for a very long to come.

So how do you prevent the feeling of being old? Decondition negative sayings and images through positive reinforcement through the subconscious mind. Eliminate crankiness, complaints, blame, criticism, and pessimism. Love life. See the good in all things. Have compassion. Be grateful.

How do you avoid the bent-over shape, slumped shoulders, and slow walking? Work out daily to strengthen the core back and abdominal muscles, the hamstrings, and the quadriceps. Walk briskly with head up, chin in, and gentle tighten the upper back muscles between the shoulder blades.

Age spots? Zap them with liquid nitrogen, laser or creams.

Retire? Don't – keep active, stay engaged in life, pursue meaning in life, and continue daily accomplishments.

Begin the deconditioning process with an open mind-set by being your true self. In a paradoxical twist, people who can learn to be themselves lose the self-centered approach to life. People in a fixed mind-set respond to people and situations by trying to be what other people expect them to be and become chronically stressed and act in a self-centered way. If people act as their true self, there is no need to be someone they convince themselves to be, which is never attainable. This leads to frustration, anger, depression, inflammation, and death at an early age.

Do you know people who are chronically angry, always complaining, blaming others, and making excuses? This is fixed mind-set thinking. These people are insecure with themselves and not willing to accept their true self. They're trying to be who someone else wants them to be, and they're angry and frustrated at themselves because they fail at measuring up to this so-called flawless other person.

Let's look at some science to see if we can live to 140. I see people with lung problems every day and have calculated how long the lungs can keep them going. It's hundreds of years. Here's the calculation. The amount of air you can blow out of your lungs is measured during the first second. This test is called the *forced expiratory volume in one second,* simplified to FEV_1, and is the single best predictor of life expectancy.

The FEV_1 value is highest at age 23 years at about 3,000 milliliters. After that, there is a naturally occurring loss of about five milliliters each year. No symptoms develop until more than 60 percent of the lung function is lost. That means shortness of breath won't develop until less than 1,000 milliliters, which won't happen for 400 years (five millimeters times 400 equals 2,000 milliliters). Decreased life expectancy doesn't occur until lung function is less than 570 milliliters – that's 486 years. Your lungs will keep you going for more than 400 years, far beyond 140 years.

Do the same calculation for the heart, kidneys, liver, and pancreas – the numbers are the same. How long can a healthy brain function? Hundreds of years. We can live to 140 years.

"What's the biggest cause of not being able to live to 140?" Scott asked.

"Inflammation," I replied. "The top causes of death have their origin in chronic inflammation, which is the underlying cause of almost all heart disease, lung disease, liver disease, kidney disease as well as diabetes, hypertension, stroke, and cancer.

The major cause of chronic inflammation is eating foods with added sugar and added salt as well as foods with processed omega-6 fats and too much saturated fats.

"There's an incredible amount of evidence that says that eating junk puts your body into an inflammatory state," says Timothy Harlan, MD, assistant professor of medicine at Tulane University School of Medicine, a former restaurateur known as "Dr. Gourmet," and author of *Just Tell Me What to Eat!* "Poor-quality foods cause inflammation," Harlan says. "Can you look older because you're eating crap? Absolutely."

Eat foods that won't harm you in the right amount, at the right time, and prepared in the right manner.

Feeling old? It's in your mind. People at 70 feel like they're old because our cultural society expects people at 70 to walk slowly, have aches and pains, and talk about their age all the time. People can feel the same way in their 60s, 50s, and even 40s. Eliminate this conditioned thinking. It's true that as age advances, people can't do something as fast or as long or as many times as they did at younger ages. But, live by the lyrics of a western song: "I'm as good once, as I ever was."

Eliminate smoking and alcohol. Limit direct sun exposure.

Manage chronic stress. It causes inflammation.

Save your joints. You know that bones will last forever, and the cartilage in the joints can last for more than 500 years. Keep a healthy weight.

Adequate sleep, daily exercise, and daily alpha-brainwave time will decrease inflammation.

Let's hear a futuristic story about Cade Grant. He's a healthy, energetic 70-year-old who had his retirement party celebration last month. He's meeting with his lifestyle planner and executive recruiter to plan his next 70 years.

"Where do I start," Cade asked his recruiter.

"You get to start from the beginning. You have 70 years to go," the planner answered enthusiastically. "Let's take your current lifestyle profile to determine if any of the 15 elements need improvement."

Cade completed his lifestyle survey by answering questions on a scale from one to five on the status of the five components of well-being and the ten health practices. He scored high with his degree of happiness, being engaged in life, accomplishments, and positive social interaction. He scored low in having meaning in his life.

"What do you need to find meaning in your life?" the lifestyle planner asked.

"I retired and need to be involved in something beyond myself," Cade answered insightfully. "I need to become involved in making people's lives better, in the community, and internationally in the world."

"Sounds good. We'll use that insight in developing your career path," the planner responded.

For the ten health practices, Cade scored high in sleep, healthy nutrition, exercise, learning something new every day, alpha-brainwave time, gratitude, and compassion. He scored low in loving life, self-healing, and being his own true self.

"You marked yourself low in enjoying life, why?"

"I'm not doing anything," Cade remarked.

"Enjoying life and the love of life is not related to activity. It's looking forward to the day filled with creativity, experiences, and talking to interesting people."

"I can't wait to start the day, see my family, meet my friends to work out, and meet the daily challenges and rewards," Cade said, "but I miss seeing my friends at work."

"I think you rated yourself too low," the planner explained. "You have an excellent positive outlook on life. Realizing you miss your friends at work means we'll use this information when launching your new career to make sure you'll be working with people."

"I scored low in self-healing because I don't know what this means. How can I use this to manage high blood pressure?" Cade asked.

"Use the general principles of self-healing, starting with learning everything you can about high blood pressure. What are the causes? What are the severity levels of hypertension? What are the treatment options? What are the complications? What is the natural course of hypertension with no medical treatment?"

"That's sound advice," Cade said, "Then what?"

"See your doctor for testing to rule out a surgical cause such as renal artery stenosis or an adrenal tumor. Review the treatment options for the different types of hypertension and review the medication options that would be best for you."

"What should I do for self-healing?" Cade asked.

"Begin with using the no-added-salt lifestyle. Do not eat any foods or drink any beverages with added sodium listed on the label," answered the planner. "Use the no-added-sugar and healthy-food-quantity lifestyle to maintain a healthy weight with a body mass index near 20."

"Sounds good. What else?" Cade asked.

"Purchase an automatic blood pressure machine at the pharmacy or online, and record your readings several times a day for a few days along with your activity and state of mind, specifically during stress," the planner said.

"I have the feeling my blood pressure is related to stress, and stress that I don't realize that I have. Could this be true?"

"Yes, a component of hypertension is related to stress, especially chronic stress, and is fundamental for managing high blood pressure."

"Maybe the answer should be obvious, but how do I manage stress?"

"Use positive conditioning through the subconscious mind in a biofeedback loop with stress-calming techniques such as deep yoga breathing, massaging your temples, and massaging the back of your neck and upper back to loosen these tight muscles. Use your blood pressure readings after doing these activities to determine if they are effective," the planner answered in detail. "You can use alpha-brainwave time. Visualize releasing tension and inflammation in the small blood vessel arteries throughout your body from head to toe."

"Can you control high blood pressure by doing these activities?"

"These activities may not cure the high blood pressure, but you may be able to manage it better," replied the planner. "And that may be good enough."

"Thanks, I'll try it," Cade said.

"Let's move on. Why did you score yourself low on being your true self?" the planner asked.

"I retired and needed to remind myself that I must continue to be my true self going forward with my new career with no blame, no excuses, no criticism, and the freedom to do what I want," Cade replied.

"That's interesting motivation, and sounds like it might work," the planner said. "Let's go forward with developing your new career and look at your online survey about work style strengths and traits."

Cade completed the 34-strengths survey, and found that his five favorite work styles included ideation, strategic, maximizer, relator, and self-assurance.

"Let's explore your preferred work styles to find alignment with your future career," the planner said.

"Sounds good," Cade replied. "Can we start with ideation?"

"Ideation means you love ideas. You're relaxed and stress-free when you're coming up with ideas, exploring ideas, and developing ideas. You find connections between disparate occurrences. For your next career, consider research and development work," explained the planner. "And, it's important to think about your subconscious desires. You enjoy ideas, but I have the impression you enjoy 'your own' ideas, so you may need to start your own company rather than work for a boss."

"You're right. I do like my own ideas, and I would prefer starting my own company, but starting a company is not for everyone and not necessary to enjoy life's work," Cade said. "If I can find a company with the executive team in line with my interests and having people-centered and community-centered leadership, that will work for me."

"Sounds good. I like your perspective," the planner said. "Let's look at strategic. This is in concert with your ideation trait. This means you can sort through clutter and find the single best solution. You see patterns where others see chaos and complexity. You select and strike."

"Yes, I enjoy that skill. It's comes natural to me without thinking," Cade said. "If the job requires thinking that causes a headache, I'm not doing it. My work needs to occur naturally without stress. It's not work, it's enjoyable," Cade added.

"You're on the right track," the planner said. "Let's explore maximizer. You strive for excellence in everything you do and everything that others do. You transform strong into extraordinary."

"Thank you for the compliment," Cade said. "There seems to be a pattern emerging. Ideation, strategic, maximizer. These traits occur naturally without stress."

"Seems like consultation work may be a good fit for you. Let's look at two more of your favorites," the planner said. "Relator is your fourth favored work-style trait. This means you prefer to develop genuine and long-term relationships."

"This trait continues to be part of the pattern," replied Cade. "And explains why I miss my friends at work. Consultation work would allow me to meet new friends. "

"Self-assurance is your fifth favorite trait," concluded the planner. "You have confidence in yourself that you can deliver. You have confidence in your conclusions and judgments. You have an aura of certainty."

"That settles it," Cade concluded. "I need to start my own consulting company or work for a consultation company in line with my interests."

"Sounds like you're heading in the right direction for your next career," the planner said.

"Before we finish, what does the 'woo' factor mean? It was listed as one of the 34 strengths."

"Woo means winning others over," the planner answered. "This means you enjoy the challenge of meeting new people and getting them to like you. Strangers are not intimidating, they're energizing. You're drawn to them. You want to know their names, ask questions, and find common interests so you can develop a conversation and build rapport."

"That sounds great – I wish I had that trait," Cade said with some envy.

"It's okay to feel that way. But, you don't need this trait. You have excellent traits you can use to build success. If needed, add "woo" people to your network and hire them for sales work," replied the planner convincingly.

"Thanks for your perspective. I have five strong traits that I can use every day with enjoyment, no stress, and productively. I will continue to utilize these strengths effectively and not spend time on the other 29 traits. They're for other people," Cade concluded wisely.

"Sounds like you've chosen a career path that's best for you and that will set you up for an exciting, creative, and adventurous 70 more years," the planner summed up with enthusiasm.

CHAPTER 20
LEVEL-10 ENERGY IS FUEL FOR LIFE

You need sustained, high-level energy to do everything you need to do – at work, with family and friends, and in the community. You need what I call Level-10 Energy. When you have Level-10 Energy you have a great day – everything goes well, you're on top of the world, nothing bothers you, and you can accomplish anything!

Level-10 Energy consists of subatomic, identical packets of energy in the universe available to you everywhere and at all times. Symbolically, these energy packets are gregarious and want to be with you and help you.

You have been using Level-10 Energy all your life at the subconscious level. You know you're using Level-10 Energy when everything is going well, when you're doing something that is important to you and has meaning, when you're doing things worth getting excited about, and when you connect and work with the people you are meant to serve.

Level-10 Energy is all around us and within us. It's positive energy that is constantly expanding, resulting in a growing universe, which means there are more positive energy particles than negative energy particles. The negative energy is a repelling energy.

Create Level-10 Energy by being engaged in life, knowing what you want, where you're going, and what you're doing at all times. Have meaning in your life by always considering the other person in a social setting and embrace positive social interaction. Getting eight hours of sleep, eating healthy, nutritious food, exercising an hour a day, learning something new, having compassion and gratitude, and spending alpha-brainwave time will create Level-10 Energy.

Stay engaged in the day for Level-10 Energy. This means no complaining, no excuses, no blame, no criticism, and no anger, which all take away from being engaged in the day. Be engaged in the moment, which means being engaged in daily activities, including your morning ritual, working out, driving, social interactions, work, eating, and even sleeping. Be engaged in the activity and process of doing things instead of thinking about problems, setbacks, or personal attacks.

Meaning in your life creates Level-10 Energy. Do something beyond yourself. Going to your child's soccer game may be time consuming and keep you away from productive work, but it has meaning in your life and in your child's life. Helping a friend move or helping a friend with bureaucratic paperwork is tedious and unpleasant, but these activities have meaning to you and to your friend. Attending a community fund-raiser may cost you time and money, but it has meaning. Helping a new hire at work may be distracting, but has meaning. Meaning in your life means it's not about you, it's about the other person. All of these activities contribute to your well-being and provide a source of Level-10 Energy.

Developing positive social interactions throughout the day is a huge source of Level-10 Energy in your work life and personal life.

For another source of Level-10 Energy, consider the Positive-to-Negative (P/N) index developed by Marcial Losada in 2004. The ratio is the number of positive statements made during conversations or discussions compared to the number of negative statements. His researchers counted positive and negative comments in the business setting. As predicted, he found that high performance teams had a P/N ratio of 5.6, medium performance teams had 1.9, and unexpected was that low performance teams had a huge negative P/N ratio of .36, or two negative comments to every positive comment.

For your work life, develop self-sustaining positive interaction among coworkers, executives, and other employees. This means actively interacting with positive responses.

In marriage, John Sottman explored Positive-to-Negative ratios among 700 newlywed couples to determine whether couples will stay together or end in divorce. He counted how many positive comments and negative comments were made during a 15-minute random conversation. The 5:1 ratio is magical. Ten years later, a 3:1 or less ratio predicted divorce with 94 percent accuracy. Negative comments are powerful. For every negative comment, neutralize them with five positive comments for successful recovery.

There are several health practices that will provide Level-10 Energy. The first one is that you need to love life. You need to want to live every day to enjoy, create meaning, and have positive social interactions.

Level-10 Energy is created by healthy nutrition, eight hours of sleep, and one hour of daily continuous exercise. Learning something new every day will create an abundance of Level-10 Energy. Spending some alpha-brainwave meditation time and practice self-healing, being grateful, and having compassion creates Level-10 Energy.

You can gain Level-10 Energy from your work. You create energy at work by focusing on positive events and interactions. You also create energy by doing work that you love and care about. Follow your passion. Love your work and you'll be good at it.

Make a concentrated effort to find your five favorite work strengths and behaviors. You like to come up with ideas. You like to work with people. You like to organize. Know your five recurrent behaviors and activities that you enjoy doing every day and keep returning to over and over through the years. Know them and study them. Take the internet 34 -strength profile and confirm your top five. As soon as you know them, align your work and job with these natural innate behaviors. You will enjoy the work. You will do better than anyone else. You will not tire of the challenges. Your passion for the work will energize your life.

Music can also give you energy. Think about it, you've listened to music that created an emotional response of happiness or love. Certain types of music can produce feel-good neurotransmitters such as endorphins and dopamine. For example, scientists gave a group of people listening to music an anti-endorphin substance and, as expected, none of them experienced an improved feeling while people *not* given the substance listening to the same music felt a *positive* feeling.

———

Let's transition to quick boosts of Level-10 Energy. Most of these are common-sense actions, but some of them may be new to you. Learn the list and use one or two of them to overcome your next low-energy moment.

Smile. A smile creates warm feelings and feel-good neurotransmitters. Smiling makes people feel happy and creates energy because other people will respond in a positive way. Laughter, especially a big hearty laugh, will give you a burst of energy.

Stand up. Surprisingly, standing will give you energy. Stand while you're talking to someone, stand while you work for a few minutes, and especially stand while you talk on the telephone. Standing triggers muscle groups for an extra boost of energy.

The strength posture. The fight and flight posture influences your conscious mind from a subconscious reflex. The fight posture of standing tall with open arms will make you feel strong while the flight posture of cowering, folded arms, and head down will make you feel weak. This has been tested by having one group assume the fight posture for several minutes and another group assuming the flight posture. A simulated job interviewer scored the fight posture people more positive than the flight posture people. Body language can influence the way you feel in positive and negative ways. Head up is good and head down is bad. Head up is strong and head down is weak.

Help someone for a burst of Level-10 Energy. This doesn't have to be dramatic. Help somebody find their car, find their papers, find a parking spot, shovel snow, organize a birthday party, make a repair, or recover from a personal setback. The simpler, the better. It's the simple step that will give you a quick burst of energy.

Compliment someone. This is easy to do. Compliment someone on their positive attitude, a job well done, providing a good answer or solution, or wearing uplifting clothes. The right compliment is two for one;

not only does it provide a quick burst of energy for you, but it also energizes the other person as well.

Make a sale or close a deal. Big or small, it'll give you energy. You've worked hard to find a client, give your pitch, respond to objections, and close. You sign the deal, shake hands, and make money. This is pure energy.

Call a positive client or a positive friend. You've had call after call, rejection after rejection. It's time to call a positive client. Just to talk. It'll give you energy.

Take a cold shower. This is how you do it. First use comfortable warm water going down your neck and back. Gradually turn the dial to cold and let it run down your spine for a few seconds. Then turn it back to warm for a few seconds. Repeat this three to five times. You'll trigger a massive energy response. Your eyes will be wide open and your skin will be tingling.

Drink water for a quick boost of energy. Find your mind wondering, developing a food craving, feeling sleepy? Drink some water.

A warm sesame oil massage can give you wonderful energy. The skin is filled with immune response cells and energy growth factors. A massage will stimulate and energize the skin and your body. Two to three minutes in the steam room will have the same effect on the skin, restoring natural healthy oils and stimulating the immune system.

Looking good will give you energy. Clothes and colors that fit your personality will give you energy. Find out what they are, talk to an expert.

There are hundreds of other sources of energy, both big and small. Discover your own. When you do, share them – it will create even more energy. Bursts of energy can keep your life vital and strong.

Create Level-10 Energy days for life. It's the feeling of being on top of the world with no worries. It's the feeling of doing anything you want without stress. It's the feeling of unlimited creativity. It's the feeling of enjoying every minute of the day. It's the best feeling in the world. It's a way of life.

Level-10 Energy according to quantum physics. It's the energy available in the universe in the form of subatomic boson energy particles.

In order to understand these energy particles, it's helpful to know how they were discovered. During the 1920s in India, physics professor Satyendra Bose was lecturing to his students about basic physics, and he asked them if they had object A and object B and two buckets, how many combinations of object A and B could be placed in each bucket? That's easy, it's four, the students answered quickly: AA, AB, BA, and BB.

"No, it's three!" exclaimed Professor Bose. The students thought he was incompetent. The lecture was published and brought ridicule from other physicists, but not from Albert Einstein. He realized it was one of the most important discoveries of the century, and it became a fundamental part of quantum physics.

Why? The students and other physicists assumed object A and object B were two different objects resulting in four combinations; however, if object A and object B were identical, there would be three. Even with this explanation, skepticism remained because physics was founded on the snowflake and sand particle theories – no two snowflakes and no two particles of sand are identical. That is true; however, for quantum physics, Bose and Einstein told the world there are subatomic energy particles in the universe that are identical. They're called *bosons*, after Bose.

Almost a century later, these bosons have been well studied and solved another enigma. What's light? It acts like a particle, and it acts like a wave, but which is it? Light consists of photons, which are energy particle bosons able to act as both particles and waves. Helium atoms are another example of bosons. They're identical and gregarious, grouping together. At near absolute-zero temperature, they flow down a glass container as expected, but have the strange behavior of flowing up too.

There are opposite energy particles in the universe that are also identical to each other but the opposite force of bosons. They're fermions named after nuclear physicist, Enrico Fermi. Instead of attracting each other and grouping together, they repel and drive each other off. These negative fermions are mandatory as they are the solidifying glue in the universe balancing out the positive bosons stabilizing the universe. However, if there were the same number of bosons as fermions, the universe would be stagnant, and since the universe is expanding, there are slightly more positive bosons than fermions.

So what's Level-10 Energy? My theory is that this is like a hologram energy in the universe. A hologram is an object that if you cut it in half, it's still whole. You can cut it into tiny pieces, and each piece contains the whole image. This is Level-10 energy, subatomic packets of that are each identical. Furthermore, taken from quantum physics, this packet of energy contains information that includes everything that has happened since the beginning of the universe, everything that's going on at this moment, and everything that will happen in the future.

Theoretical uses of Level-10 Energy based on quantum physics. Level-10 Energy can be used to solve problems, heal, fend off negative energy, and explain synchronicity and serendipity.

Use Level-10 Energy for solving problems and healing. These packets of energy are identical and each one of them has an infinite amount of information. Learn to communicate with these particles and use the information to your benefit. Use this information for solving problems and healing. You do this through your subconscious mind while in alpha- and theta-brainwave states.

Negative energy has been used throughout history to hurt people, as seen through ancient psychic practices used to cause pain. This is only effective, however, if the other person believes. The same is true for the healing power of Level-10 Energy. This can be used for the healing process.

Fend off negative energy. There is almost an equal amount of negative energy fermion packets in the universe, and they're everywhere. You know people who dwell in the negative Level-10 Energy world, and you've had negative Level-10 Energy used against you. These negative forces exist in the form of criticism, blame, jealousy, shame, resentment, fear, doubt, guilt, gloom, sadness, insecurity, and anger.

Fortunately, there are more positive energy packets than negative packets because the universe is expanding instead of shrinking, positive instead of negative. So you have more than enough positive energy to counteract all negative energy. Send out Level-10 Energy to counter and neutralize the negative forces, thoughts, and words that other people are sending your way.

Level-10 Energy can explain synchronicity and serendipity. Synchronicity occurs when two seemingly unrelated events come together to create a common outcome. You pass by a bookstore to browse, and the book you need falls off the shelf. You're looking for a parking spot during holiday season, and as you arrive at your store, a car pulls out just for you. If Level-10 Energy is involved, synchronicity is going have a good outcome. Serendipity is better – it's a happy coincidence or miracle discovery.

There are many instances of seemingly unrelated events that none-theless are united. For example, have you ever thought about a childhood friend and when the phone rings, it's that very person? Or, how a mother knows that her child is in danger and rushes to a distant scene to save her child? Or why scientists in two different countries make the same discovery simultaneously?

Take the example of thinking about your college roommate and an email arrives a few minutes later, and it's your roommate. How does this happen? Is this by statistical chance? You have 300 thoughts per minute, which would be 4.5 billion thoughts in 30 years, which means the other person also has 4.5 billion thoughts. The chance of both of these thoughts occurring at the same time is unlikely, nearly impossible. What about transporting these thoughts by brainwaves? No, brainwaves are too short and too slow. They cannot travel thousands of miles.

Level-10 Energy is the answer. Here's how it works. It's a five-component Einstein thought experiment.

First, Level-10 Energy consists of subatomic packets of pure energy, each one identical, and they're gregarious. They love to be near each other. These energy packets make up 70 percent of the universe and are expanding at an astonishing speed. That's 46,000 miles per second and getting faster. That's a huge amount of Level-10 Energy.

Second, these Level-10 Energy packets are like a hologram. Each one contains all of the information in the universe from the past, present, and future. Therefore, as you think about your friend or roommate, each Level-10 Energy packet in the universe already has the matching thought. There's no lag time because time is not involved. These tiny packets of energy are in every cell of the body, including the brain and the source of thought. Therefore, your thoughts are instantly available.

Third, your thought has a unique Level-10 Energy configuration.

Fourth, there is a complementary replica of this thought from the other person in each of these holographic Level-10 Energy packets.

Fifth, these two configurations meld together causing the synchronicity or serendipity outcome. It's like pieces of a puzzle with two separate pieces of Level-10 Energy forming a single piece.

The implications of this thought experiment are exciting. Your friend calling or the two scientists from separate laboratories creating the same result are random. But, what if we could learn to create these occurrences? We've been told there are opportunities all around us. This is true, but how do you connect with them? If you're single, you know that your lifelong spouse is somewhere, but how do you make the connection? You know there is an answer to a problem, how do you find it?

How do these thoughts meld together? Seeking out the corresponding thought by searching is impossible as there are infinite thoughts available in the Level-10 Energy pool. Try this: create the alpha-brainwave or theta-brainwave state, visualize the complementary thought, and merge the connection with your mind. If people can learn to do this, the ability could change the way humans behave and interact. Imagine what thinking and communication will be like 200 years from now. That's Level-10 Energy.

CHAPTER 21
PEOPLE-CENTERED
LEADERSHIP

Good leadership requires a boundless amount of energy. What makes a good leader? Making decisions is at top of the list. Other traits include positive social communication, commitment, confidence, persistence, creativity, integrity, and for the entrepreneur, funding and team building. These traits can be learned, and for best results, practiced in a self-sustaining and self-maintaining way.

There are several types of leadership styles. Laissez-faire is hands-off and often leads to confusion. Autocratic leaders are a thing of the past; they are quick and effective but leave a trail of destruction. Participative leaders go by the book, leading by a fear-based reward and punishment system. Transformational leaders are creative and challenge teams to work toward change.

Most leadership types are counterproductive and egocentric. Become a *people-centered leader* – an inspirational leader who cares about people.

Making decisions is not only the job of the leader, but also other executives and everyone in the organization. You make thousands of decisions every day. Should I get up or sleep longer? Which clothes to wear? Should I eat something for breakfast? What should it be? How long will it take? How much work will it be? You've made 50 to 100 decisions before you even start the day or go to work.

For leadership to be effective, decisions must be made fast. It's not about being right or wrong. It's about making a decision. If it's right, you can move on. If it's wrong, fix it.

Making no decision or delaying the decision stops action and bringing the organization to a standstill. Nothing is done. Former secretary of state Colin Powell often talked about how indecision can lead to confusion and loss of thousands of lives. The right decision moves the business in a successful direction, and a wrong decision moves the business to fix it.

Consider decision fatigue. A specific brain energy is needed for making these thousands of daily decisions. This is the adenosine energy that is used up by the end of the day. This is why you might make bad decisions at night such as eating too much, drinking too much, or buying something too expensive.

If you're a decision energy saver, this explains why you may be annoyed when friends and coworkers ask you what they should eat, what they should drink, what clothes they should wear, whether they should go to a meeting or not, or other personal choices. Each answer uses up a small amount of the adenosine energy, especially if you have to give a reason for your answer. Furthermore, often the person already knows their decision and is making conversation, ignoring your answer. This can be mitigated by the other person saying that's a great decision, I like what you said, thanks. It neutralizes the negative energy used and restores or even exceeds the depleted decision energy.

Professor Ryan Hamilton at Emory University summarizes his decision-making research into the four "R's" that can be used for how we make decisions in our lives as well as how we make buying decisions for goods and services.

Reference points matter as in the reference point that is used to make a decision. Is this an accurate reference point based on important elements of the issue or an inaccurate reference point based on an authority opinion, celebrity or brand name.

Reasons are important. People make decisions based on reasons which is good as long as the reasons are sound and relevant to the issue. The answer should not be based on whether asked a positive question or negative question, because of the physical environment or other non-related reasons.

Resources matter. People have limited amount of energy for attention and self-control. People make good decisions if they devote sufficient cognitive resources for making a decision. However, if the information is too complex or people have exhausted their decision energy, people use habitual responses or easy heuristics not related to the issue or value of the product or service.

Replacement is important. People have many workarounds when they are presented with difficult tasks, and will replace these hard tasks with easy tasks. Chose a CEO who is decisive, positive communicator, creative, and innovative? This may be too difficult to determine, so people may use easier ways such as making the choice because the person is friendly or may look like a CEO.

Positive communication is interacting with people in ways that result in a positive feeling by all participants. Life is about emotions, and feeling good as many times during any given day results in a productive day. Talking with people in an organization creates a positive feeling for both the leader and the team members. Talking to coworkers, clerks, and restaurant staff in a positive manner increases personal energy and feel-good transmitters.

Commitment means always doing what you say you will do 100 percent of the time, with no exceptions. You say yes to a meeting, to a dinner party, to helping someone, or to volunteering. Do it, even if a better offer comes along or you change your mind. There is no problem saying no to the offer. If you don't want to do something or have a conflict, say no – say no to free tickets, no to an invitation, and even no to a request for help. This is meaningful for both participants, since saying yes and then not showing up is bad for everyone. This makes you feel bad and makes the other person doubt your character. Say no. If you say yes, do whatever it takes to do it.

Confidence is needed to be a good leader. Do you like to follow someone who is weak and has no confidence in a decision, plan, or project? You feel bad when you have no confidence in yourself. Increasing your self-esteem is not enough. We have great self-esteem when everything is going well, but when things get tough, self-esteem jumps ship and abandons us.

Use compassion for yourself. This never lets you down. Confidence comes from how much we like ourselves. Learn to be your true self for full confidence.

Persistence is fundamental for continuing success in life. Author Dr. Angela Duckworth uses the term *grit* to describe perseverance and passion. Grit consists of courage, which often means eliminating the fear of failure; endurance and follow-through; and resilience – the optimism and confidence required to bounce back from failure. It's not concentrating on winning, it's concentrating on doing your individual best. Grit also means not quitting because the task or project is too hard or someone told you to quit or that you're not good enough. Stop only because you have completed the job or reached your goal.

Creativity is the spice of life. This means using your mind to solve day-to-day problems. Using your mind to make things happen, to create projects for the community, to create products, to create solutions, create businesses, and to create enjoyment for yourself and for your family. Increase your creative ability, and you will improve your life and everyone else's too.

Integrity and honesty are the foundations of a good leader. This is obvious for an executive or boss, but even more important is being honest with yourself at a private level. No exaggerations, no convenient forgetting, and no stretching the truth. Always be honest with yourself. No lies. No rationalizing. In many situations, the raw truth will be painful, and sometimes extremely painful, but recovery will occur. The ancient saying is correct: The truth *will* set you free.

Funding and team building are essential for entrepreneurs starting a business.

These are the attributes of a people-centered leader. How do you draw on them in a sustainable manner? Use the five components of well-being and the ten health practices. Common elements include healthy nutrition, eight hours of sleep every night, one hour of continuous exercise daily, alpha-brainwave time, and stress management through self-healing.

These healthy lifestyle habits also sustain and replenish brain decision-making energy. In addition, your decision-making skills and ability to make decisions fast are improved when you learn something new every day and when you're engaged in life at all times, know what you want, where you're going, and what you're doing.

Positive social communication can be improved through being engaged in life, having meaning in your life, enjoying life, having compassion, and being grateful.

Self-confidence is elevated by happiness, being engaged in life, having meaning in life, daily accomplishments, learning something new every day, having compassion, being grateful, and most importantly, being your own true self.

Persistence requires having meaning in your life, daily accomplishments, alpha-brainwave time, and being grateful.

Creativity comes from being happy, being engaged in life, having meaning in life, and learning something new every day. Being your true self is fundamental for creativity as all other considerations become a distraction taking away valuable creativity time. For creativity, it's helpful to sometimes take the prefrontal cortex judgmental center offline through alpha-brainwave time or an hour of continuous exercise.

Integrity requires being engaged in life at all times, having meaning in life, being grateful, and especially having compassion for yourself and others. You must be your true self at all times. Integrity also requires eight hours of sleep, healthy nutrition, and an hour of continuous exercise.

Funding and team building for the entrepreneur requires maximizing all five components of well-being and all of the ten health practices for success.

CHAPTER 22
HARD WORK
AND AMERICAN
ENTREPRENEURSHIP

America owns entrepreneurship. It's the driving force of success. The company builders of the late 19th century and early 20th century include Carnegie, Rockefeller, Edison, and Ford. The Wright brothers. Our modern builders include Bill Gates and Elon Musk.

The American spirit of independence and the right balance of restrictive regulations to protect businesses combined with incentives to allow entrepreneurial businesses to thrive have created boundless opportunities in this country.

Americans love hard work. It feels good. It contributes to society. It provides income with freedom to spend. Tocqueville wrote that America is where everyone works to earn a living and labor is held in honor.

Let's talk about some of today's American hard workers. Johnnie from a national television cable company. We needed to upgrade our equipment. Johnnie arrived at our home on time with clean clothes. He put paper covering on his boots so he wouldn't get our rugs dirty. He installed the new equipment and got it working without complaining or blaming us for anything. He explained ten new features in detail and in a pleasant way. He went on his way – this is an American working hard, not complaining, not blaming the customer for anything, completing 100 percent of the job and doing a good job the first time.

Here's another example. The owner of a fast-food restaurant at a service plaza facility along an interstate highway near Boston is a hardworking American who proudly displays pictures of himself and his family along with pictures of his awards for outstanding service. The site is immaculate without a loose piece of paper or trash anywhere. There are decorations throughout the facility celebrating the current holiday. Everything is clean. Like the owner, the people working behind the counters are pleasant and are dressed nicely. The owner also manages several other locations along the way, which all have the same spirit of cleanliness and hard work. The owner is proud to be a hard worker and everyone visiting the facilities benefits.

Our enclosed upstairs shower needed tile re-grouting and cleaning. Theo arrived in his white van with his company name painted on the outside. He greeted us with a big smile and went to work. It was hot, grimy work in a tight space. We offered water and a fan, but he said he was fine. He smiled and kept working, sweat pouring from his forehead. He had no complaints about the heat, the confined work area, or the caustic chemicals and harsh brushes. He finished the job and cleaned the area, returning the bathroom to pristine condition. His invoice was reasonable and exactly as he had previously quoted. On the way out to his truck, he proudly showed us pictures of his family now in America who he works so hard to support. Theo is an excellent example of a hardworking entrepreneur who doesn't complain, blame others, or make excuses.

Nike cofounder, Phil (Buck) Knight illustrates three entrepreneurial lessons about pursuing your passion, being persistent, and dealing with competition.

Buck was a track athlete for the University of Oregon and, like millions of other 25-year-olds, he had no idea what he wanted to do. But, he did know one thing. He liked sneakers – he was obsessed with sneakers.

He earned his master's degree from Stanford and, again not knowing what he wanted to do for a living, he moved home. Phil decided he needed to explore the world. In Japan he stopped by a running shoe company and asked to be their US distributor. He persuaded them to ship him some shoes.

Months went by without receiving any word. Phil had returned home and needed to work. He had an informational interview with a family friend who was a company CEO. Phil was thinking that the CEO would tell him to start his own company. Nope, he said to become a CPA, a lifetime job opportunity. Not an exciting career for him, but Phil took his advice because he didn't have a better alternative. He took the courses and began his job search.

Then the shoes arrived, and he received the exclusive rights to sell the Japanese shoes in the US. This was the greatest day of his life. He loved shoes. He smelled them, felt the lacings and admired the soles. He put them on. He stacked them up in the basement.

Phil ventured out with a huge smile and fired-up determination to sell them at sporting goods stores who would welcome him with open arms and be excited about the opportunity to sell a new brand of running shoes. As you and I might have expected, he received rejection after rejection. No one needed another running shoe.

So the entrepreneurial spirit provided him with the idea of loading them up in the trunk of his green Valiant and go to track meets all over the Northwest. The running sneakers were a huge hit. They felt good, runners loved them, and they were cheap. He sold all of them and sent in an order for 1,000. He was happy. He was doing what he wanted to do and following his passion for shoes. He was a "shoe dog," which became the name of his book.

Then he received the letter from the East Coast – cease and desist! The letter was from the so-called rightful owner of the US rights to sell these Japanese shoes. This began a series hurdles and roadblocks that develop along the way to success. Phil mastered each one of them to go on to develop a world-class company, and demonstrated that the entrepreneurial components of persistence and never quitting.

Phil tells an important story about how to deal with competition in daily life and in the business world. Everyone knows that competition is good, the better the competition, the better you do. But, it's not the competition that makes you do well, instead it's "not" thinking about the competition and "forgetting" the competition. Think about and concentrate on doing the best you can do and then squeezing out more.

When Phil was a runner athlete at Oregon, he competed against world-class athletes who would later go on to the Olympics. He considered himself an above-average athlete, but not in this league. He had no chance competing against these runners. At first, it was all he could think about the night before a race, the morning of a race, and at the starting line. But, he quickly learned that having these thoughts took up valuable space in his mind that would lead to defeat along with poor personal times.

Phil changed. He stopped thinking about the competitors. He never let the thought of these competitors in his mind. He focused his thoughts on doing the best he could do, planning his speed, gaining speed at the end, and going all-out over the finish line.

This approach applies to business. Learn about your competitors. What they're doing. Where they're going. And forget. Concentrate on doing the best you can do. If you've been rejected, fired, or treated in a unjust way, you have to leave these feelings behind to free your mind so that you can concentrate on doing the best that you can going forward, presenting yourself and your pitch with care, confidence, and success. Any emotional anger baggage on your mind is lethal and will derail chances of a successful outcome. Phil learned to beat the competition by forgetting the competition.

Living in South Africa, Elon Musk loved to read during his childhood and was often made fun of by the bullies in his classes because of his love of knowledge. During his 20s, Elon came to the US, lured by the American spirit of independence and the right balance of governmental restrictive regulations to protect businesses so they could thrive.

He immediately recognized an opportunity to develop a needed payment system on the internet and cofounded PayPal to satisfy this need. A basic precept of entrepreneurship – developing an innovative solution for a neglected need.

From there, Elon created a spaceship factory. Success this time occurred because of another entrepreneurial tenet – do something no one else does. Instead of building rocket engines from past designs, Elon built engines designed by his own engineers from "bottom up." Furthermore, all materials to build the engines came from America, not using thousands of parts imported from other regions of the world that were traditionally used to build rocket engines. This saved millions of dollars because of time saved and because of the reduction of a multitude of administrative and document work, damaged materials, transportation expenses, and poorly designed items.

Elon also broke from tradition by designing his spaceships to take off from and land at the same location. He did things that no one else did. He built spaceships from original design, using American components, and built a spaceship that could take off from and land in the same place.

Elon went on to build a factory for an electric car and used the same entrepreneurial style – original designs by his engineers and using all American parts. He also built a solar panel factory. Hyperloop and Mars are the next stops on his entrepreneurial train.

For every one of these out-of-the world success stories, there are hundreds and thousands of stories that don't yield financial success.

I will tell you about my entrepreneurial experiences to illustrate the most common outcome of developing a startup. None have mine have been a major financial success, yet they have been exhilarating and filled with meaning, accomplishments, working with extraordinary people, and most of the time, enjoyable. Whatever you do, don't quit your day job. It's the thrill and rewards of the *process* that provide the impetus to try again.

I began with what you need to do. Do something you're passionate about. For me, it's the health and medical industry. In medicine, there are three discoveries to be made: finding the cause of a disease, finding a disease, and discovering a treatment. While in medical school in New Orleans, I discovered a new cause of a disease – it was a parasite that caused the lung fluke disease in Colombia, South America. Later, during my lung fellowship training program in Boston, I discovered a lung disease called bronchiolitis obliterans organizing pneumonia (BOOP).

After this second discovery, I wanted to discover the third one – a new treatment. This took the form of three requirements. First, it was going to be a social population treatment, one that would improve the lives of people throughout the world. Second, it was going to be commercial-based. Third, the discovery had to be financially successful so the financial gains could be used to build new services and products to improve people's lives.

I quickly realized I had no skills in sales, finance, business, or starting a company. Medical school is to learn how to diagnose and treat disease. Therefore, I began my quest to learn.

I started with Zig Ziglar, who could teach me how to sell. The first thing Zig said was to "respond" and "not react" to problems. Stay calm and think rather than use up negative energy reacting emotionally. Look at the good things in people and the fighting stops.

There are five reasons why someone won't buy what you're selling – no need, no desire, no money, no hurry, and no trust. You need to sell something people want, not what they need. You have to create the desire. Your integrity will allow people to trust you.

If you are selling to a company, talk with the decision maker. This results in a 45 percent closing rate compared to eight percent for a fill-in person. Take the reasons why a person can't buy and use them for reasons why they must buy.

Don't be brought down by negative thinking. If the country is in recession, decide that you're not going to join in. You'll have a better chance to succeed because half of the competition is fighting the recession by cutting costs and not developing new products. You're the opposite, you take all the business that was lost.

Zig gives ten selling tips. (1) Project a positive demeanor, sell before you go. The new sales kid story, he went to the wrong address but sold the biggest order ever because he had sold it before going there. (2) Assume the buyer is going to buy the product when you make your pitch. (3) Physical appearance needs to be appropriate for the sale. (4) Enthusiasm for life and for the sale. You may lose one sale because of too much enthusiasm, but you'll lose 15 because of not enough. (5) Ask a question that most people will answer with a yes response. If it's a yes, you have a sale. If not, you will obtain information to make the sale. Examples include: Have you sold yourself? Should I tell you more? Do you see this is good for your health? (6) Listen with your eyes. Watch the body language. If someone says no but they're stroking the plush surface or salivating, they're saying yes. (7) Persistence is fundamental. Years ago, an Australian encyclopedia salesman spent six hours in the home of a mother who said, "Thank you, thank you for taking the time to show me how these books can help my son." (8) Talk about an upcoming event, a new product, a new sale, or a new price increase. (9) Use inducement – persuade or influence someone to buy with an inducement. (10) Be sincere. Selling is a transference of feeling. If someone feels the same way about your product that you do, they will buy. Transfer your enthusiasm about a product to someone.

Use a powerful opening line, not "I have a program to sell you," but "I have a program to increase your sales."

Every product or service has six objections. Be prepared for them – they're conditions, not objections.

The old sales model was like a battle between the salesperson and the customer, a fight for who would win. There are four components of a successful sales model. Building trust and listening is 40 percent of the equation. Identifying the needs of the prospect as they relate to your product is 30 percent, and giving your pitch about what the person needs is 20 percent of the process. Gaining confirmation and commitment to action is the final ten percent of the equation.

Prospecting is part of the sales cycle. Learn to ask questions. Find the problems that your product or service can solve. Ask open-ended questions about how much the prospect knows about your company and what the customer is doing in this area. What is your overall problem and specific problem?

Don't talk about benefits customers don't want or need. "Teaching takes place with your words, but learning takes place with your silences," reports best-selling author Brian Tracy.

A good way to deal with objections is Brian Tracy's "feel, felt, and found" method. I understand how you "feel" about the price, color, texture, etc., and others "felt" the same way about the price, but this is what they "found": they were so happy with the product they bought more. Use emotions to sell.

Closing the sale is sometimes so traumatic that half of the time, people don't even try to close; however, customers expect you to ask for the close and are at a loss if you don't ask. There are hundreds of types of closes and new ones develop every year. One of my favorites is the *puppy-dog close.*

"Go ahead take the puppy home for the night; if it doesn't work out, bring the puppy back." These are preceded by trial closes.

The *invitational close* is "Do you have any further questions? Does this make sense so far? Well then, if you like it, why don't you give it a try?" The *assumption close* is if there are no further questions, the next step is to package it, deliver it. The *alternative close* gives choices: "Which would you prefer, red or blue?" The *incremental close* is making a small decision first, then on to the bigger decisions, getting three yesses. The *authorization close* is when the prospect has no further questions, get out the contract, show them where to sign with a check mark (not an *X*), and ask for their authorization to sign. The *order sheet close* is taking out the order sheet and beginning to fill it out. "What is the correct spelling of your last name? What is the correct address?" Pause. There are hundreds of closes.

When it comes to persuasion, Jay Conger says to use the following techniques in order of importance: examples, analogies, and stories. Use emotion as the most powerful method of persuasion.

Harvey Mackay says don't try too hard. Sometimes it's not needed. For example, two bars lost their licenses because of late hours. They appeared before the city council. One had a high-priced lawyer who threatened to sue the city; they threw the book at him. The other represented himself with street clothes and an apology; they gave him a warning.

Harvey Mackay's 15 negotiating rules: (1) Never accept anything immediately. (2) Don't negotiate with yourself; make an offer and get a counteroffer. (3) Never cut a deal with someone who has to go back to the boss to get approval because they get two shots to your one. (4) If you can't say yes, it's no. (5) Even if it looks nonnegotiable, it probably isn't; call the bluff. (6) Do your homework. (7) Practice and rehearse. (8) Beware the late dealer; they may just be trying to make you believe they don't care about making the deal. (9) Be nice. If you can't be nice, have someone else do the job so you don't ruin the deal. (10) A deal can be made when both parties see their benefits. (11) Set a scene, help the other side visualize the benefits. (12) Don't talk about your business where people can overhear you. (13) Watch the game films – debrief after a session. (14) No one is going to show you their hole card; you have to figure out what they are really after. The given reason is always false, therefore eliminate it. (15) Always let the other side talk first.

Kerry Johnson talks about three types of buyers. Determine which type someone is and speak to them in terms that will help persuade them to buy.

For *visual* people, say, "I see how you feel – others saw the same thing, but this is what they found" and "They were happy."

For *auditory* people, say, "I hear you, it sounds good to me," "I like the sound of that," and "I hear what you're saying – others heard the same thing, but this is what they found."

For *kinesthetic* people, say, "It feels right to me," "It feels good to me," "I like the way that feels," "I understand how you feel about the price – others felt the same way, but this is what they found," and "They were so happy they bought more."

Helpful "laws of power" for sales by Robert Greene include always say less than necessary; guard your reputation with your life; win through your actions, not through argument; do not build a fortress to protect yourself because isolation is dangerous; continually re-create yourself; despise the free lunch; don't appear too perfect; and don't go past your sale by knowing when to stop. Most importantly, plan all the way to the end.

Robert Cialdini writes about six sales principles of persuasion, including reciprocity, liking, social proof, authority, scarcity, and consistency. These principles can be useful in getting a yes from your customer. For example, someone doing a clipboard survey at a busy street corner had a 20 percent yield, but when the surveyor first asked people if they considered themselves helpful, all answered yes and there was a fourfold increase in completing the survey, up to a 78 percent yield.

Another person who was selling a new soft drink was asking for email addresses and received a 20 percent response rate. But, after asking people if they were adventurous – and 97 percent said yes – the yield increased to 75 percent.

For television ads associated with thrillers, advertise for groups by showing general features of the product, but for romantic shows, advertise for individuals by showing individual features of the product.

It's helpful to learn about the "O" waves in the brain abbreviated from the "orienting" response of the brain. These O waves are triggered by change in the environment. This discovery came to light when scientists who worked on the Pavlov dog experiments wanted to show other scientists and the press how the dogs behaved after a bell goes off. The dogs were conditioned to salivate after hearing a bell go off because in the past the dogs were given food after the bell rang. But the dogs did not behave as they had in previous experiments. Why not? Because the dogs were *distracted by a change in environment.* The new people watching triggered O waves that overrode the learned bell response.

This happens to us all the time. You're not losing your memory when you can't find your keys or cell phone; you were distracted by a change in the environment and the O waves displaced the memory of your keys and cell phone location.

In selling and advertising, TV cuts are more important than clips. Cut to something you want to sell because the "O" waves will override the past action and people will buy the product.

The words you use can be important in selling products and services. If you're in the health business, use "nonviolent" words. Use *information points* not *bullet points; approach* a problem, don't *attack* it; and *outpace* other companies, don't *beat* them. If you're an airline pilot, don't use "death" words. Say *destination,* not *final destination* and *gate,* not *terminal.*

Use achievement words and images to sell to runners and athletes. In your workplace environment and your office, use success and action images, and update frequently. If you're doing a questionnaire or survey, say, "I would like your *advice,*" rather than *opinion.*

After learning about sales, I went on to take business courses about finance, business structure, and business models. I spent several week-long sessions learning about marketing and advertising. All of this took several years.

Prepared with this information, I began my quest to build a company that would create products and services to improve the lives of people all over the world. But before this, I needed to learn about **living in the world of rejections.**

After receiving 25 one-page rejection letters from medical schools throughout the United States, on the second day of medical school, I was thrilled to hear Professor Knight's magical words, "We've had a cancellation. You're in."

This was the biggest thrill of my life and was the end of rejections. There was one success after another nonstop for years and years.

Until I began the startup life. Then, rejections became a daily staple.

My first series of rejections began when I developed a quality management system for hospitals that would provide continuous improvement in medical care. I was so excited about this system that I wanted to publish a book to tell the world about it. I wrote the book and immediately found a literary agent in Boston. Just as immediately, she contacted me a week later and said that it had been rejected by all of the publishers she worked with.

Not fazed and not deterred, I wrote a massive book proposal and sent it along with sample chapters by FedEx to 50 publishers. I received nothing from 45 of them and 5 rejections letters from the others. This book was never published. Welcome to the world of rejections – now rejections were becoming painful. They began to hurt.

Yet, my enthusiasm for hospital quality management remained constant, and I wanted to develop a related software program. But I couldn't do this alone. I needed help. I needed a partner. This led me to the streets of Boston and the new businesses springing up in Cambridge, which in turn led me to one rejection after another for three years.

My friend told me that a colleague of ours sold a medical publication for $140 million. I had not known this vast amount of money existed in the medical publication business. It gave me the idea of publishing 250 books, each one about a rare disease that could potentially help millions of people throughout the world who could improve their lives by learning about their rare disease, how it's diagnosed, the treatment options, and how to manage the disease.

I would begin by publishing my book about BOOP, the rare lung disease that I discovered. Expecting ten percent of the people with the disease to buy the book, I was prepared for selling 50 books per day. The reality was that no books were sold in the first 30 days and only one book was sold the next month. Sales were similar for the rest of the year. This effort of a rare disease medical publishing company startup was abandoned.

During my sales training years, I learned that I had needed to accept rejection in order to be successful. "Another rejection means you're closer to the sale," I was told. "Learn to love rejections because it means you're making sales calls," I was also told.

Rejections dominated my next attempts at building products and services to improve people's lives. They included a companion drug/genomic testing product, a transportable ER and urgent care center using steel shipping containers as a building platform, and a dietary supplement for air pollution.

I had a session in Jack Canfield's home where I learned about rejection when 15 of us were asked to request something from each other. Mine was: "Would you hire me as a spokesperson for your company?" The other person was to say "no" nine times and "yes" the tenth time. After several rejections, you no longer take the exchange personally or emotionally. This exercise was helpful as rejection became more mechanical without thinking, taking out the negative emotional feeling.

Rejection in real time. Recently, a Hollywood agency asked if I wanted to make a movie out of one of my books. These were health books and not particularly exciting material for a movie. So, I wrote a medical thriller that was partially based on an experience in an ER that I had during medical school in New Orleans. The book could serve as a movie script.

It's a fictional book intended for light reading during summer break on the beach. I needed to find a literary agent who could sell the manuscript to a publisher for publication and sale. At first, I recorded these attempts, thinking I would have success after a few emails, but this was not to be.

Sunday evening, I completed the final editing changes and started my search for a literary agent. I found nine pages listing 336 literary agents who were willing to accept an email proposal. I reviewed each entry, narrowing the list to 25 agents located in New York City. I further limited this list to seven by researching their websites and publication successes.

The next day, Monday, I developed a general email pitch after refining many drafts, and I wrote a personalized email to each of the seven literary agents, enclosing the chapter one introduction. I pushed "Send" to all seven at 11 in the morning. At 1:00 p.m. I received the magical response from an agent in New York, "Thanks so much for writing! I'd love to read the full manuscript."

After the hundreds of rejections during the past year, this email made me feel so wonderful, but it was a preliminary response and full acceptance as my literary agent depended on reading the entire manuscript.

It's now Thursday morning, and that wonderful feeling was quickly replaced with doubt as time had gone by without any word, going through the day and night checking emails with this feeling of persistent doubt in my stomach mixed with the feeling of hope for a positive response.

In the meantime, I received a personal response from one agent who chose to pass and another agent who would review the request and get back to me in eight to ten weeks. At least these were responses, much improved conversion rate. Nothing from the other four.

So today still Thursday, I sent the four a checking-in email by forwarding the original email. I was nervous about sending the New York agent an email because I didn't want to bother him, but I need to know if he received the full manuscript. He quickly answered in the affirmative, and I asked if we could meet Monday in New York in his office. He declined and said we could meet in May, and he would send me a note with his thoughts about the book. The stress of the unknown continued.

Now Friday, nothing from the four checking-in emails. I sent a fresh group of emails saying that I will be in New York Monday and would love to see them. I received a response, no, "out of town," but it was a response. Three to go.

Monday morning in New York City. I sent out two emails to LA talent agencies located in New York saying I was thinking about developing a movie from the book, hoping this would spark an interest. Nothing, no response. I sent a third email saying I was in New York and could meet in the office during the day – nothing, no response.

Tuesday, 9 p.m., received the rejection email from the initial New York agent who responded positively to my first email within a couple of hours. The book is too commercial, and the agent was searching for in-depth character development for book club discussions.

This ended my week-long rejection episode for trying to find a New York literary agent. Summary included review of 336 agents, in-depth review of 35 agents, selection of seven to contact, 25 emails, six rejections, one pending review, and requiring ten hours of dedicated work plus the elation from one response, the stress from waiting for an answer, the stress from a non-commitment, and the final blow of total rejection.

In success stories, this is where you read that out of nowhere, a call comes from the best literary agent in New York: "We just repaired a flawed computer glitch that scrambled your book, and after reading the manuscript, it's so good, we're putting you on the fast track for publication." You read about these stories over and over, but you have to know these are one in a million. My end result is the most common not only for me but for everyone else in the rejection business of startups.

At this stage you ask yourself why this is not successful. I'm talking about a book, but the same is true as an entrepreneur starting with a product or service – why isn't this successful?

You start with objective reasons. Timing is wrong, medical thrillers are not popular right now. The book business is dying; no one is buying books. Literary agents are too busy to take on a new book. There's not enough money in publishing a medical thriller.

You continue listing objective reasons, searching for something you can do something about, but soon you deteriorate to personal reasons. Who am I kidding? I can't write. I'm not smart enough. I can't sell anything. The writing is boring, not deep enough. I'm not interesting enough, and the self-deprecating list goes on, leading to negative thinking and thoughts of ending the quest.

But, you've chosen to be in the entrepreneurial startup world, and you quickly shrug off this type of thinking and go on to round two.

It's Thursday, round two, day five. I found seven more top agents from a list of 25 literary agents, including one from Boston. Emails sent 9:25 a.m. and one FedEx, three responses with a good conversion rate – two will review in six weeks and one out of town. Thursday, one week later, seven "checking-in" emails sent with no response.

There is time and an emotional roller coaster associated with this work. First, do the research about the literary agent to find out background and interests. Second, write the email choosing each word, phrase, and sentence to persuade, sell, cajole, and get a positive answer. Third, sending the email, which is associated with a positive result – complete with visualizing meeting with the person, seeing the office, talking about the deal, and seeing the book on the *New York Times* bestseller list. All this requires time, energy, emotional feelings, and stress.

The stress is self-imposed from trying to find the right information and developing the right words to get an acceptance. A single word can make the difference between receiving a reply and not receiving a reply. Receiving no responses results in frustration. Receiving rejections is painful. Sometimes, you go through the five stages of grief for a few minutes or even up to 48 hours. But, you persist, on to round three.

Thursday, day 12, review of the list of 25 yielded seven new literary agents in New York and emails were sent as well as four additional checking-in emails sent to previous agencies. Friday, five FedEx packages were sent to five agencies willing to receive snail mail. This took two hours of work with individualized cover letters, and 20 pages of the manuscript. Now, money has been spent, which will require one hundred book sales to cover the cost. By Tuesday, all five of the FedEx packages had been received, but not a single response. Sunday, received an email rejection, "Not for us, thanks."

It's on to round four, day 24, and a change of tactics. Send the manuscript directly to a publisher, bypassing the literary agent. After two hours of research, five publishers were found and five emails were sent. No response from any of them.

It's day 41, round five, and a new hurdle developed – a new title was needed. I found out a book with the identical title was published the previous year. Ten days later, four rejections arrived by email. "I'm going to pass and it doesn't fit into my list." In the meantime, I came up with a new title as well as an introductory story modified from my own experience in a hospital ER. Successful books are based on personal experiences as these are always unique.

Thursday, round six, and day 61. I sent 14 emails to past agents who had not responded with the new title and new introduction, and received three rejections within 48 hours. After two months of rejections, the emotional response once again developed as frustration and confusion as to why there has been no success. Tuesday, sent out 13 new emails to literary agents among all 336 listed, now totaling 36 contacts and two more rejections received. Wednesday, day 67, 16 emails to new agents including one in California. Monday, day 72, 18 emails to agents in New York and Los Angeles. I was in New York for three days and sent ten emails saying, "I'm in New York and can talk in your office," and not a single response. By Wednesday, day 81, I had now reached a decision stage about abandoning the project since this book is not going to strike a fit with any of the literary agents.

But, I didn't quit, on to round seven, day 94. If I could rewrite the query subject line and rewrite the first three paragraphs, someone would respond. I resubmitted 39 emails with a "checking in" subject line, and sent 14 emails to new agents, for a total of 89 literary agents. I received one request for an abstract, which was rejected after review. By Wednesday, I had sent out emails to 94 literary agents and 188 additional checking-in emails, and had received 54 rejections by email and no acceptances.

It's now day 110, round eight. I had abandoned the project for several days, but found several new literary agents. I wrote three emails to publishers and 12 new emails to New York literary agents, for a total of 110 inquiries.

It's Wednesday, the project has been abandoned after six months at day 187. The effort included 350 emails, FedEx packages, and telephone calls to 110 literary agents with 43 documented rejections. The opportunity cost included hundreds of hours of my time with a monetary value of thousands of dollars and no book publication.

Was the process worth it? No, and this effort was not enjoyable. Yet this is the entrepreneurial world of rejection and likely common among those taking the risk of being the boss. It's not recommended for everyone.

The steps toward making a discovery are the same as starting a company. During a pathology lecture in the second year of medical school, I saw the words *bronchiolitis obliterans* in the textbook and asked, "What's bronchiolitis obliterans?"

"It's a mystery," replied the professor.

This was the first step of discovery and is the first step for a startup. It's an ancient saying by now – find your passion. For me it was bronchiolitis obliterans. For Buck Knight at Nike it was shoes. For you, it may be finance, law, software, or one of thousands of other endeavors.

The next step is research and study. Several years later during my post–medical school training, I searched a database of 5,000 individuals who had lung disease and found 100 of them labeled as "bronchiolitis obliterans." This is the second step for a startup: narrow your search to a list of 25 to 50 specific opportunities within your general interest.

There is an intermediate step required after developing your passion and before beginning the work. Something else happened to me during the four to six years between seeing the words in the textbook and starting the work. I developed confidence in myself.

Without self-confidence, I never would have gone on to the next step. As a second-year medical student, my mind-set was closed. I had been rejected for admission by medical school after medical school because of lower grades and lower MCAT scores than students given acceptances. So I felt that everyone was smarter than me and, furthermore, I felt that I needed to prove that I was good enough to be in the class. My mind was so filled with these thoughts, there was no space for thinking about doing something on my own.

Yet, during the last two years of medical school and a grueling medical internship at Harlem Hospital in New York City, I developed confidence in myself and abandoned the negative thinking and the need to be someone else. This newfound confidence soared when I was considered an international expert in tuberculosis through my national service work at the Centers for Disease Control in Atlanta.

This confidence brought me to Boston, where I was surrounded by intelligent and successful doctors, and rather than feeling inferior, I held my own and took advantage of their teaching. I had no feelings about anyone being smarter than me, and I had nothing to prove. This created an open mind-set and the realization that I alone could accomplish what I wished to do.

To start a business, you need to go through this period of growth by gaining self-confidence and accepting your true self. It's a mandatory requirement to be able to manage and survive the huge obstacles that will develop beginning day one and every day during the life of the company. In addition, to thrive, it's important to maximize the 15 lifestyle elements in this book to your benefit and to maintain them for the energy required to succeed.

After doing the initial screening, it's time to go to the third step. I obtained all the information available for each one of the 100 patients. I made a spreadsheet that contained all the clinical features, the chest X-ray findings, lung function test results, treatment, and the microscopic cellular reaction of each patient.

For your startup, analyze each of the 25 to 50 subcategories of your passion with a score of one to ten. From here, develop a spread-sheet with the opportunities on the left, and across the top add ease of entry, complexity of the topic, time involved, cost, potential income for you, how much you would enjoy the topic, will people want the product or service (they may need the product, but not necessarily want the product), and, most importantly, can it be a profitable busi-ness or is it only a good idea? The answers can be given on a scale of one to five.

Now to step four, look for a pattern in the spreadsheet. This is what I found, there were 50 patients that had a lung disease process that was described during the early 1900s and was well known. But, there were 50 patients that had a disease that had never been described. Instead of limited to small airways, this process was inflammation that involved both the terminal region of the small bronchiole airways and the lung itself, which was called bronchiolitis obliterans organizing pneumonia, or BOOP for short. This was a breakthrough discovery that would pre-vent prolonged illness and save lives!

For your startup, it's time to review the spreadsheet and search for a pattern with the highest scores for you. Select the product or service and go forward.

Now the discovery has been made or the business has been selected, and it's time for the next extremely difficult and complex step. Gaining acceptance.

I showed the chest X-rays of a representative case to the professor.

"What's this? This doesn't mean anything," grumbled the professor, shaking his jowls. "I need you to work on my project."

Intimidated and deflated, I returned to my assigned work. But, I continued working on my own work after hours and on the weekends.

My friend asked me, "Why is the light on in the fifth floor of the blue building in the middle of the night?"

"I'm working," I responded, keeping my activity to myself.

Several months later, I showed the professor a different case, and was sent away with the same admonishment.

But, this is where perseverance for entrepreneurs is a must. After several more months, I showed him a third case, saying in a forceful and overexcited voice, "I have 50 just like this one."

"Why didn't you tell me earlier?" the professor roared, this time realizing the significance of the discovery.

There are several lessons from this step. You must learn to manage rejection as everyone, including your friends, your family, and investors, are going to tell you that your idea is not new, not innovative, and not a business. You also need dogged persistence as you will need to pitch your idea over and over and continuously develop improvements in your pitch as you go.

The final step in the discovery process is finding a way to get the world to know about it. For BOOP, I was fortunate enough to associate myself with one of the most well-known professors in the world and who was connected throughout the globe. With the help of the professor, I wrote up my findings for these 50 cases. The study was published in the *New England Journal of Medicine,* which was the most widely read and prestigious medical journal in the world. That launched this discovery throughout the globe, and I was asked to talk about BOOP all over the planet.

To this day, physicians in the lung department of hospitals in any region in the world know about the "BOOP doctor." There have been more than 1,000 new reports about BOOP, and the discovery has prevented suffering and saved lives throughout the world.

So the final stage of building a successful startup is finding someone or a partnership with such stature that they will be able to help you launch the company. This is no small feat as the number of people or partners is limited, the competition to find these people is intense, and coming up with a novel way to hook up with these people is difficult. Persist and succeed.

The twists and turns of entrepreneurship provide the excitement and exhilaration of potential success. If you decide to start your own business, enjoy the journey.

CHAPTER 23
BUSINESS ONE-LINERS

"In a business or social setting, it's always about the other person."

– Gary Epler

Take profit first. You're starting a business. Money comes in from a sale or service, take 10 percent as profit first and pay expenses with what's left over. This way, you'll make money from the beginning. After all, you are the most important employee and you should be paid for doing the work. The old model of starving entrepreneurs is gone. Paying expenses first and taking profit after all the money has been spent leads to stress, frustration, and failure.

Pixar films are not finished, they're released.

Give the good news in individual amounts. Give bad news in one big amount. People are happier if they win a $25 lottery ticket and a $50 lottery ticket the same day rather than winning a $75 lottery ticket in one day. However, people are sadder if they receive a $25 tax bill and a $50 tax bill the same day rather than a single $75 tax bill.

People like flat rates better than pay by play.

Make decisions and make decisions fast. This is from my friend, K, who has a billion-dollar whey-manufacturing company. After earning a master's degree in chemistry from the University of Florida, he was surprised to find that people who had prestigious degrees from Harvard, Yale, and Stanford would work for him and would listen to him. Why would anyone listen to someone without the intellectual capacity of these brainy people? He soon realized it's because he made decisions. He had to make decisions minute-by-minute throughout the day. He learned to make them instantly with decisiveness and conviction because he realized it's about making the decision, not the issue or the content. If the decision is correct, he, his employees, and the company will move forward. If the decision is wrong, he and his employees will fix it. Make decisions fast; not making decisions leads to failure.

Use the worm's-eye view. Trying to solve problems from the bird's-eye view blurs facts that are needed to find solutions. Go to the street and ask questions. For example: a basket maker in India made only pennies per basket, even though each one sold for a thousand times more than that, and it took a very long time to make each basket. It was not until someone knocked on people's doors and asked questions that the injustice came to light and a more equitable system was developed, improving the standard of living for these basket makers.

Break down the end product into small pieces. For successful product development, start with small pieces, work on them, and release them to the next step. Find problems and solve them as you go. There is no reason for a committee or anyone to develop a detailed plan to find the problems and the solutions before beginning because almost all problems encountered cannot be identified in advance. Committee meetings, decision making, and document writing take hours of time that could be used for developing the product. Start small, build a small piece, fix a problem that develops, and move on.

Improve every aspect of your business in a small way to become the best in your industry. This means analyzing every detail of your business and then developing a method of improving each one of these details in some small way. For example, the British cycling team wanted to become world competitive. They hired a person to analyze and identify every part of winning a cycling race from the bike, to the rider, to the training, and to the timing and location of the event. They hired an additional person to develop a way to improve each one of these. They discovered there was one hour between the prequalifying event and the qualifying event, so they filled every minute with activities that could lead them to victory, such as stretching, eating a nutritious snack, mental training, and tuning up the bike. The team went on to win international events.

To improve your performance in running marathons, playing tennis or golf, or Zumba, in addition to practicing the sport, strengthen your body every day – including the core, biceps, triceps, hamstrings, and quads. Also, always remember to hydrate, eat healthy, nutritious food, and get enough sleep.

Use the subconscious mind for sales and persuasion. All decisions are made by the subconscious mind. Functional MRI (fMRI) portrait studies have shown that the sequence of decision-making events always begins in the subconscious mind, which in turn sends the signals to the conscious mind. This sequence helps us perform our daily living tasks such as brushing our teeth, walking, and driving a car; however, the subconscious mind also makes all of our important behavior decisions, good or bad.

Therefore, for sales and persuasion, you need to communicate with the subconscious mind, not the conscious mind, which means it's not about the words or language, it's about creating conditioning through images, sound, or touch. This is the reason Oren Klaff was so successful at raising a billion dollars in capital for entrepreneurs. He explains how in his book, *Pitch Anything.*

"Talk to the croc brain," he reveals. This is the primitive and ancient emotional crocodile brain located in the subcortical region of our brain. This croc brain only responds to emotions that result in two outcomes, pleasure or protection. Interactions that cause fear, mistrust, or giving too much information mean protection, which means shutting down the system and fleeing.

To gain and maintain the attention of this croc brain, you need to elicit comfort. If you're careful, you can also use the fear component without losing the connection. For example, Klaff activates the pleasure component of the croc brain by creating desire by offering a reward, and activates the fear and protection component with tension by showing the stakes will be high if the deal is lost.

This emotional selling has been used to sell goods at the local marketplace for more than 5,000 years. And now, it's used by the advertising

GARY R. EPLER, M.D.

business and salespeople on a daily basis. Sell to the subconscious through images, sounds, and touch.

Learn about these effects on the subconscious brain so that you can avoid developing opinions and making decisions based on negative subconscious conditioning. The knowledge that the subconscious mind makes all behavioral decisions explains why brainwashing through negative conditioning can be so effective. Association of negative emotional images with a certain group of people or events over and over develops a dislike or, even worse, hatred toward this group of people or events. For buying products or making social decisions, we need to learn when to recognize this negative conditioning so that we can analyze the situation through our own decision-making process.

Leaders will be those who empower others. Bill Gates talks about leaders of the future. Successful leaders are going to be people-centered leaders. These leaders are healthy and fit. They are engaged in life. They have meaning in life. They commit to positive social interaction. They empower everyone around them.

AI is software writing software. Data in, insight out. Jensen Huang, CEO of Nvidia uses the term artificial intelligence (AI) to include all the sub-artificial intelligent names such as machine learning, deep learning, and artificial neural networks. Huang says that AI means to teach computers to do something. Put data in and get an answer out. Train the data to generate software. AI training AI to develop AI. Data scientists develop training data strategies and develop software with a training strategy that will write software by itself. Build an intelligent machine – data comes in, action is taken, and products develop.

Network and ask questions. Networking results in making connections that lead to business success. This means genuinely connecting with people because it's enjoyable and an opportunity for learning. This does not mean connecting with people for making money or obtaining free advice.

Talk to people in your business about their work life. How did they become interested in what they're doing? What project are they currently working on? What is the biggest problem they're dealing with now? The answers will help you learn about your business, and you in turn may be able to help them with a part of their business or send them a referral.

Sometimes, you'll hear a random phrase or one-liner unrelated to the business conversation that will be helpful to you that you'll remember forever. You'll apply this to your everyday life and work. You'll tell other people about this new insight. And, you might come up with a random one-liner that will improve the lives of other people.

CHAPTER 24
HOW TO USE THIS BOOK

Use this book as a guide for the health and fitness lifestyle. Feeling low, no energy, and having a nonproductive day? Review the five components of well-being and the ten health practices. One or more of them will fix the problem, kick-start your positive feelings, and get you back on track. Copy pages, learn the 15 elements, make a list, and develop a way to review them at any time or in any place. Feeling guilty, sad, out-of-sorts, down-in-the-dumps? Review them for repair. They will take care you for a long, long time.

ABOUT THE AUTHOR

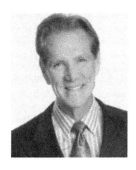

Dr. Gary Epler is an internationally known Harvard Medical School professor and thought leader in health, fitness, nutrition, and people-centered leadership. He is an award-winning author and has impacted the lives of people throughout the world through his speaking engagements, books, and teaching. He has been called upon by individuals from around the globe who have a rare lung disease that he discovered. Dr. Epler is a successful entrepreneur. He has been founder and CEO of three companies that include a biotech company, a nutraceutical company, and the current medical consulting company. He is a sought-after speaker, addressing audiences about health, fitness, nutrition, and leadership.

Dr. Epler has been recognized yearly since 1994 in *The Best Doctors in America.* He believes personalized health empowers people. He has written four health books in the critically acclaimed "You're the Boss" series about people taking charge of their health including *Manage Your Disease, BOOP, Asthma,* and *Food: You're the Boss.* Dr. Epler's recent book, *Fuel for Life: Level-10 Energy,* is about living a high-energy life filled with enjoyment and creativity.

Dr. Epler discovered the treatable lung disorder bronchiolitis obliterans organizing pneumonia (BOOP). He found a new parasite in South America, chronicled the nutritional needs of North African children, and managed the tuberculosis refugee program in Southeast Asia. Dr. Epler was Chief of Medicine at the New England Baptist Hospital for 15 years. In addition to conducting clinical and research work, Dr. Epler strives to educate. He has written more than 110 scientific reports and given hundreds of seminars and lectures throughout the world. He became editor-in-chief of an internet-based educational program in critical care and pulmonary medicine offered by the American College of Chest Physicians. *Business Week* acclaimed him for his develop-ment of e-health educational programs that enable patients to manage their health and disease. Dr. Epler was recognized as one of *Boston Magazine*'s "Top Doctors in Town."

Dr. Epler has run several marathons including Boston, New York, and Paris, where he proposed to his wife; and for their first anniversary, they ran the original Greek marathon together. He delivered the twentieth baby from a mother who named the baby after him. He's been one of the Boston Celtics team doctors. He has taught medicine throughout the world and was fortunate enough to save a dying infant in South America from an overwhelming parasitic infection by using the sap from a fig tree. He saved a baby who choked on a donut during a little league baseball game that he was coaching. He is a radio and television personality. He is a Hollywood screenwriter and has written a medical thriller movie, medical drama TV show, and a lifestyle reality TV show. He is active in the community. He coached soccer, basketball, hockey, baseball, and club baseball at Boston College. He lives in the Boston area with his wife, Joan.

Contacting Dr. Gary Epler

Address:	Epler Health, Inc.
	888 Worcester Street, Suite 205
	Wellesley, MA 02482
Email:	gepler@comcast.net
Website:	www.eplerhealth.com
Facebook:	https://www.facebook.com/eplerhealth?fref=ts
Twitter:	https://twitter.com/EplerHealth
LinkedIn:	https://www.linkedin.com/in/gary-epler-8736a610/

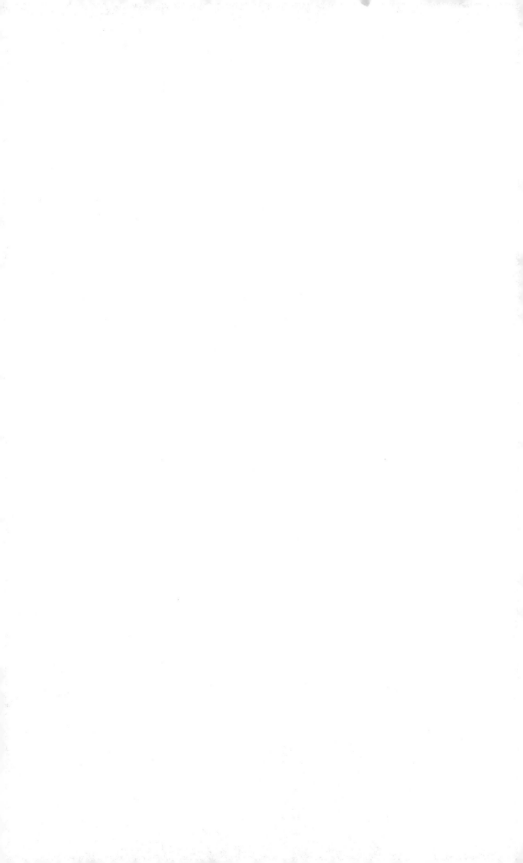

CPSIA information can be obtained
at www.ICGtesting.com
Printed in the USA
LVHW080525150319
610767LV00025B/411/P